The Unvaccinated Child.

A Treatment Guide for Parents and Caregivers

1st Edition

Judith Thompson, ND

Eli Camp, ND, DHANP

With Contributions by

Judith Boice, ND, LAc, FABNO

Vital Health Publishing

© 2017 by Judith Thompson and Eli Camp

Published in 2017 by Vital Health Publishing, LLC

Vital Health Publishing, LLC

Norman, Oklahoma

Printed in the United States of America

Book Design by Antonio Conway

ISBN: 978-0-9995165-1-5

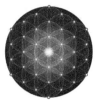

Vital Health Publishing

Visit us on the web at https://www.vitalhealthpublishing.com

Acknowledgements

We start our acknowledgements by thanking those leaders and pioneers whose dedication and commitment helped build and preserve the field of natural therapeutics and ensured the existence of vitalistic naturopathic medicine as we know it today: Hahnemann, Priessnitz, Kent, Dewey, Felter, Spitler, Wendel, Coulter, Hering, Lindlahr, Lust, Bastyr, Mitchell and Ellingsworth. In our journey of writing this book, there were many modern day teachers who have taught, mentored and inspired us to practice vitalism: Jim Sensenig, ND, Jared Zeff, ND, Letitia Dick-Kronenberg, ND, Thomas Kruzel, ND, Mona Morstein, ND, Stephen Messer, ND, Rick Kirschner, ND, Deborah Brammer, ND, Farra Swan, ND, Durr Elmore, ND, Nora Tallman, ND, CNM, Catherine Schaefer, ND, CNM, Richard Barrett, ND, Jill Stansbury, ND, Kevin Spelman, PhD, RH(AHG), and Robert Broadwell, ND. We are thankful for the time and effort of current day practitioners who have written books that we referenced in the writing of this book and that we use in clinical practice: Roger Morrison, MD, DHt, Prof. George Vithoulkas, Andre Saine, ND, Wade Boyle, ND, Russell Marz, ND, Joseph Pizzorno, ND, Michael Murray, ND, Mary Bove, MD, Robert Sears, MD, FAAP, Rosemary Gladstar, Kerry Bone, Simon Mills, and Stephen Buhner. We are incredibly grateful to Judith Boice, ND, LAc, FABNO for her expertise and contributions on essential oils. We are thankful for and could not have written this book without the experience gained through our work with hundreds of patients who were willing to place their trust in us and share our faith in the incredible healing power of nature. We finish with appreciation and thankfulness for our families who supported and encouraged us every step of the way.

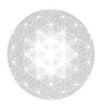

The Unvaccinated Child:
A Treatment Guide for Parents and Caregivers

Forward

You have in your hands a compendium of brilliance for raising healthy, strong, bright-eyed children. I wish to congratulate Dr. Judith Thompson, ND and Dr. Eli Camp, ND, DHANP, for writing this much-needed resource for families.

There is no need to poison our children's blood streams with toxins in the name of "prevention" when the real prevention to illness is a healthy immune system. As we are exposed to more bacteria and viruses our immune system strengthens with the experience of the previous encounter. This will then allow us to fend off chronic illnesses, degenerative diseases and cancer as we age. We do a disservice to our children if we do not allow their immune systems to encounter the common infectious diseases of the human race.

Infectious diseases are regularly treated and healed using natural principles such as fasting a fever, hydrotherapy, homeopathy, herbal medicine and other methods that support the body's wisdom. Over the last 30 years as a practicing naturopath and as a daughter of a naturopath, I have treated or have seen treated, thousands of children (and adults) that have developed these contagious diseases. The sickest of these folks are routinely the ones who had the full schedule of immunizations. Even with the most severe cases of measles or pertussis, by using these basic principles of health and healing as outlined in this text, the children have healed quickly and without harm or lasting effects.

If you have vaccinated your child, you will still want to have this information at hand. If your child becomes ill you will have a starting place to begin supporting the natural healing process which is what will heal the illness no matter what approach you take. All medicine only works to cure an illness if it supports the body in bringing the metabolic function to a higher level. If the approach given to the child is suppressive, then the condition of the body's health can only worsen. We CAN treat contagious diseases with gentle medicine that is strong, fast-acting and uncomplicated. So, let us strive to nurture the vitality of the child's body, strengthen the circulation and digestion, empower the immune system and, in doing so, let us all raise healthy children.

Dr. Letitia Dick-Kronenberg, ND

INTRODUCTION

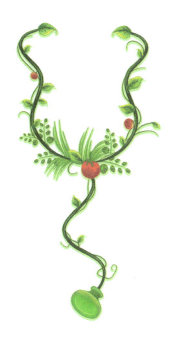

When we were first in practice, the number of parents who told us they did not want to vaccinate their children was low. They didn't want anyone to know they weren't vaccinating, but, they desperately wanted and needed medical support in order to know they were doing the right things to keep their children healthy. They suffered in silence, not telling friends, family members or medical providers that they had chosen to do something different than the conventional standard of care. Fearing ostracization from their families and communities, they didn't know that more parents were slowly making the same decision and quietly coming to us for help.

Over the years, the numbers of parents looking for information—statistics, risk factors and overall support—has grown exponentially.[1] They are becoming more aware of potential risks and want to minimize them by proactively and naturally maintaining their children's health. As naturopathic doctors, we are trained in optimizing health regardless of vaccination status, and are therefore their ideal health care practitioners. These parents feel safe and confident with the information we provide. They trust us because they know we have education in nutrition, herbal medicine, homeopathy, immune system development, physiology and children's health.[2]

Since many of these conditions are not as prevalent as they used to be, parents' and caregivers' ability to restore health when faced with these diseases has been lost. Neither parents nor medical providers are aware that these conditions can easily be managed through natural means. Our intent is to provide education and resources for parents who have decided it is best for their family not to vaccinate their children.

A Note to Parents That Have Vaccinated Their Children

If your child has had some injections and not others, this book can still be a helpful guide, especially those sections that discuss how to support your child's immune system through specific illnesses. If your child is in full compliance with the current vaccination schedule, they too can benefit from this book, since statistics show that children in full compliance have the highest rates of actual illness.[3] Whether a child is not vaccinated, partly vaccinated or fully vaccinated, this book provides parents the information to keep children in the best health possible.

A Note on Methodology

The statistical and disease presentation information in this book comes from public information readily available through public health organizations such as the National Institutes for Health (NIH), Centers for Disease Control (CDC) and the World Health Organization (WHO) as well as medical texts and journals from the US National Library of Medicine. Treatment guidelines come from interviews with doctors that have been in practice over thirty years (some have over forty or fifty years of practice experience or were mentored by doctors that were in practice in the mid-20th century when these conditions were commonly seen).

We have also consulted research from new publications about the effectiveness of vitamins, minerals, herbs, homeopathic remedies and other natural therapies, as well as reviews of older literature available from doctors that were treating these conditions at the time when they were most prevalent, i.e. before vaccinations were available. Some of the treatments discussed are from Eclectic doctors, doctors from the late 19th and early 20th century who used herbs, homeopathic remedies and minerals to help the body heal.

By compiling information from different sources including books, medical journals, public health records, medical professionals and historical documents, we aim to bring all available information together to assist parents and caregivers in working with these conditions, and to include as many of the natural therapeutics known to re-establish health.

Finally, a number of the protocols discussed come directly from our clinical practices, working with hundreds of children using vitalistic naturopathic modalities of healing.

What It Means to be "Unvaccinated"

For the purposes of this book, "unvaccinated" refers to children that have not had injections of bacteria, viruses or toxins (including the chemicals associated with injections). Children exposed to contagious diseases naturally (through being out and about in the world) are still considered unvaccinated.

Parents may choose not to vaccinate their children for a variety of reasons. A large percentage are motivated by religious and philosophical beliefs, while others are concerned about possible health risks associated with vaccinating. We are not saying to vaccinate or not to vaccinate children, but for parents that choose not to vaccinate, there are requirements of caring for children that accompany that choice.

A decision not to vaccinate carries with it the responsibility of being proactive in caring for a child. There are necessary actions to implement to keep a child healthy and able to ward off and recover from illness. First, parents must provide a healthy diet of fresh foods, clean water adequate exercise, proper rest and emotional support. Second, time must be spent with children. When sick, it takes time to nurture a child through illness, and this could mean keeping a child at home for days or weeks if there is an outbreak of an illness. In daily life, keeping a child healthy could be taking the time to prepare homemade food for every meal and not eating out. Not vaccinating may require making the decision to not allow a child to eat birthday cake and ice cream at a friend's party. It could mean exclusion from attending specific schools or summer camp programs that will not accept unvaccinated children.

These are difficult but necessary decisions for parents to make as a child is growing up and wanting to participate in different educational, sport or social events. Nevertheless, there are private schools that accept unvaccinated children and some state health departments that will provide vaccination exemption forms for attendance in public schools. There are also numerous support groups to help parents navigate through their decision.

A Brief History of Germs

When the germ theory was established in the 1860s[4], people began viewing disease as resulting from exposure to particular microorganisms.[5] This perspective suggested that a person was perpetually at the mercy of microorganisms, which could cause death without any level of protection. As a result, people were frightened to be around anyone that was sick for fear they might catch something.

Concurrently, there was another theory of health and illness known as the terrain theory. The terrain theory[6] held that the internal environment of a person's body (the health of their cells and tissues) determined her or his susceptibility to illness.[7] If a person had good metabolism, strong immunity and normal detoxification, that person was not as susceptible to disease.

Interestingly, prior to the existence of the germ theory, from the time of Hippocrates (and prior to Hippocrates, as seen in traditional Chinese medicine and Ayurvedic medicine), it was widely believed that imbalances in the body caused illness and disease. If unclean air or miasma (an old term describing unhealthy elements) affected the body, it was because the body had a susceptibility or vulnerability for illness.[8]

Oral traditions tell us the concept of increasing immunity has been a part of Indigenous practices around the world. The medicine people of varying indigenous tribes such as the Cherokee[9] exposed community members to contagious diseases by sharing a sick person's blankets or placing the sputum of a sick person on a healthy person's skin or wounded area. This small exposure to illness, although it initially may have made the person sick, was believed to ultimately help the person increase immunity and stay healthy. Today, this concept is alive by parents that have their children play with other children with chickenpox to enhance natural immunity through natural exposure. The critical piece to note here is that those people are exposed through natural routes of exposure—i.e. skin and respiratory airways, not through unnatural exposure via muscle tissue via an injection—promoting a natural immune response.

The other important factor to consider is that families with known contagious illnesses also quarantined themselves, thereby stopping the spread of illness while allowing the natural development and healing of illness.

1 As of the writing of this book, the Centers for Disease Control (CDC) has changed how they distribute this type of information. Whereas they used to give numbers of diagnosed contagious diseases, they now only give percentages on their front pages. (This is concerning because in the cases of some contagious disease that have very low numbers. For example, rubella with less than 10 cases per year, a 100% increase would mean 10 more people in the country were diagnosed with it but that type of percentage can scare the public into accepting mandatory vaccinations.) Currently, much statistical data is either unavailable or buried within public records.

2 For clarity, when the word "we" is mentioned in the book, it refers to the authors of the book.

3 Center for Disease Control and Prevention. "2015 Final Pertussis Surveillance Report". https://www.cdc.gov/pertussis/downloads/pertuss-surv-report-2015. pdf (accessed Feb 15, 2017)

4 Brought to Life Exploring the History of Medicine. "Germ Theory." http:// broughttolife.sciencemuseum.org.uk//broughttolife/techniques/germtheory (accessed March 23rd, 2017)

5 Louis Pasteur's research established the germ theory.

6 The terrain theory was initiated by Claude Bernard (1813-1878) and continued with the work of Anton Bechamp (1816-1908).

7 Henry, Derek. "Germ vs Terrain Theory – Which Do We Adopt To Be Healthy?" Natural News Blogs. https://www.naturalnewsblogs.com/germ-vs-terrain-theory-adopt-healthy (accessed March 23, 2017)

8 Encyclopedia.com. Biomedicine and Health: The Germ Theory of Disease. http://www.encyclopedia.com/science/science-magazines/biomedicine-and-health-germ-theory-disease (accessed March 23, 2017)

9 Eli Camp, ND, DHANP

PART I
Immunology and Prevention

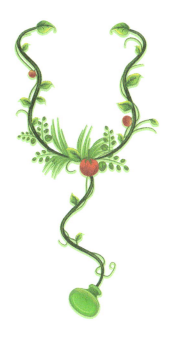

You may have heard "Prevention is the best medicine," or "An ounce of prevention is worth a pound of cure." These phrases speak to the value of staying healthy. There are habits to practice every day to keep ourselves and our loved ones in good health. Keeping up these habits, although they may require time and effort, promote quality of life and allow people to pursue the things they love. The body knows how to be and stay healthy. It's up to us to help it stay that way.

Chapter 1:
An Overview of Vitalism

Vitalism is the understanding that there are biological, chemical and physical forces at work in living beings, as well as an energetic component that goes beyond biochemical and physical forces. This energetic component, although it does not have a direct definition in Western terms, is known as *Qi* in Chinese medicine and *prana* in Ayurvedic medicine. In naturopathic medicine, it is known as the *Vis* or the *Vital Force*. Together, these biological, chemical and energetic forces create vitality and drive normal and healthy functioning within the body.

Vitalism views the body as a living organism rather than a machine with replaceable parts. Our bodies are much more than the sum of their parts. When damaged, a machine does not have the ability to repair itself. In contrast, our bodies have an innate intelligence that guides healing and restoration. Vitalism recognizes and engages this intelligence or "body wisdom" to speed recovery from illness and build even greater levels of health.

Vis Medicatrix Naturae

Taking a vitalistic and naturopathic perspective when it comes to health allows for optimal body function. When one looks to nature, the inherent capacity for healing is observed. Wounds heal, fractures mend and new growth appears. This is one of the principles of naturopathic medicine, the *Vis Medicatrix Naturae* (the healing power of nature). Left to its own processes, the body's default state is toward health. Vitalistically and naturopathically, the aim is to support that process with natural remedies. In nature, the resources with which the body can heal are abundant. Those items contain their own vitality which, in turn, nourish our bodies, minds and spirits.

The Vis

When looking at a person's level of health, there are specific traits that show vitality. As humans, we know it when we experience it or see it in another person. Those characteristics or traits are signs of the vitality that flows through and in us. For example, we may look for features like:

- bright eyes
- clear skin
- a robust complexion
- strong nails and hair
- toned muscles
- enduring energy
- sound sleep
- strong digestion
- daily bowel movements
- a stable, predominantly positive mood

These are all examples of a strong *Vis*. When a person is sick these characteristics are not present or have been weakened. This calls for strengthening of the *Vis*. Part 2 discusses ways to stay healthy and keep the *Vis* strong, thereby preventing illness.

Chapter 2:
Naturopathic Foundations of Health

There are foundational steps to being healthy, preventing illness and promoting the *Vis*. They start with keeping the digestive system running, maintaining the nervous system in a calm state and supporting the muscular system. Promoting wellness, and thereby immunity, requires that all body systems are functioning at their best. When the foundational steps are covered, the *Vis* is enhanced and the immune system is strengthened.

Immunity

Often when parents come for a visit they are looking for a "natural way" to treat the immune system. They are surprised to learn that creating an optimally functioning immune system is more than simply taking a natural substance. Optimal immune function results from building healthy body systems, interacting with nature such as playing outdoors and reducing environmental toxins. It also includes making lifestyle choices such as incorporating a healthy diet, getting proper sleep and providing a peaceful, safe, fun and supportive home life.

Physical immunity starts in the gut. Along the lining of the digestive tract lies the gut associated lymphoid tissue (GALT), which is a part of the immune system that protects the body from foreign invaders in the digestive tract. Within the GALT are cells called Peyer's patches which regulate bacteria in the gut by creating an inhospitable environment for unfriendly bacteria and allowing healthy bacteria to remain in the small intestine. These cells are our first line defense from toxins and pathogens that come into our body from the outside. Studies show that human fetuses have Peyer's patches developed by thirty weeks of gestation.[1]

Another way our immune system develops and stays strong is by exposure to microorganisms. Humans have a symbiotic relationship with trillions of microbes that support and work with our immune system. Every time a person comes across a new bacteria, it will induce the innate immune system (for example, there will be an increase in natural killer cell activity and more macrophages will be released). The immune system will create more B cells (antibodies) by stimulating adaptive immune responses or support normal function (by destroying and eliminating foreign organisms).

Mothers that breastfeed their babies are passing on their own microbiota, as well as cytokines (immune signalling cells), immune cells, metabolites and IgA (a type of antibody), via breast milk. One of the ways breast milk is protective is by maternal IgA not allowing microbial attachment. That is in addition to expanding the number of friendly bacteria in the newborn.[2]

Ultimately, the more exposed a person is to microorganisms, the more robustly the immune system develops. Studies have shown that overexposure to antibiotics, poor diet and lack of probiotics in our food have lead to higher rates of inflammation[3] and can negatively affect the developing gut.[4]

Digestion

Good digestion is the cornerstone of health allowing absorption of critically important nutrients while eliminating toxins from metabolic waste. Digestion encompasses numerous organs and many different biochemical reactions. If the digestive tract is viewed as a tube with one opening being the mouth and the other being the anus, it is seen that there is a function for every part of the digestive tract.

Chew Your Food

In our mouths, saliva and enzymes are released that help us breakdown food. In our fast-paced world, many people have forgotten the importance of chewing, even though it is an important part of digestion. The more we chew our food, the less strain we put on our stomach, liver, gallbladder and pancreas to release hydrochloric acid, pancreatic enzymes, bile and other digestive juices.

Train Your Digestive System

Having ½ teaspoon of apple cider vinegar before meals can promote further breakdown of food by increasing digestive secretions. This is an excellent method for training the body to do what it knows how to do when digestion has not been optimal. As nutrients are absorbed in the small intestines and water is reabsorbed in the large intestines, the leftover material bulks up and leaves the body if there is an adequate amount of fiber and water in the diet. Supporting these steps as food travels through the body is the best way to maintain a healthy gut.

Nervous System

The nervous system is closely tied to the digestive system because foods eaten go directly toward forming body tissue. The brain itself is made up of fatty tissue and nerve fibers have a fatty layer around them called the myelin sheath. The myelin sheath promotes normal nerve function, allowing nerve fibers to travel at optimal speeds. Eating adequate amounts of healthy fats builds healthy brain and nervous system tissues.

Diet

As one of the primary staples of good health, food creates biochemical reactions that either support health or detract from it. Different foods provide vitamins, minerals, antioxidants, healthy fats, bioflavonoids and fiber that all add to normal body function and strong immunity. Interestingly, one of the biggest risk factors for contraction of illness and severity of disease is malnutrition. In fact, the CDC states this repeatedly when discussing prevalence of disease severity for many contagious illnesses. Keeping in mind how important our digestive system is in maintaining overall health, focusing on the critical nutrients that will maintain optimal digestive function is the way to ensure absorption of nutrients.

Vegetables

Vegetables provide phytonutrients that enhance immunity, maintain normal removal of waste products and enhance digestion and absorption of nutrients. Many green leafy vegetables like collards, kale, mustard greens and swiss chard are high in B vitamins and mineral content. Cruciferous vegetables like broccoli, cauliflower, cabbage and Brussel sprouts help keep the liver filtering and detoxifying. They also tend to be high in folate, vitamin A and magnesium. Many root vegetables provide high amounts of vitamin A, potassium and calcium. Many children find sweet potatoes, acorn squash and turnips palatable if introduced to them at an early age.

Fruits

Fruits are high in antioxidants, fiber and phytonutrients, all of which provide high vitamin C value to enhance immune function. Fruits like blueberries, blackberries and raspberries are low on the glycemic index scale, meaning they raise blood sugar levels the least after consuming them, making them a healthy choice for fruit. Apples and pears are also good options since they have higher fiber content.

With those benefits in mind, remember, not all fruits are equal. The sugar content in some fruits is so high that it can throw off the balance of microflora in your child's digestive system. High sugar fruits can feed yeast and create an imbalance in the digestive system. Bananas, mangos, peaches, apricots, nectarines, dates and figs all fall into this high sugar category.

Protein

From skin, hair, collagen, joints, muscles and nerve fiber, protein (in the form of amino acids and peptides) makes up a majority of the human body tissues. It's important to consume adequate amounts of protein to maintain healthy regeneration of new tissues. There are different sources of protein that can meet a child's needs.

- ◆ **Vegetarian sources of protein**

  Vegetarian options for proteins include beans, nuts and seeds. Of these choices, beans like lentils, black beans and lima beans provide the highest amounts of protein. They contain ample protein for a small child. As kids grow, some children like to add meat to their diets, while others don't. The choice not to eat meat may last a short time, or it may be a lifelong preference. It's okay for some children to be vegetarian; it simply requires that parents pay more attention to their child's protein intake. Vegetarian sources of protein provide enough nutritional value to meet a growing child's needs.

- ◆ **Animal sources of protein**

  If your child does want to eat meat, focusing on the quality of meat is the most important component. Lean meats that are hormone and antibiotic free (cage-free and grass-fed, if applicable) provide higher nutritional content. Keeping the intake of excess hormones and antibiotics to a minimum supports a child's normal development.

Healthy Fats

Children eating diets high in unsaturated fats (as in avocado), monounsaturated fats (such as olive oil), polyunsaturated fats (such as olive oil) and some healthy saturated fats (such as coconut oil), have strong and focused brain function.[5] Eating nuts and seeds, once their digestive system can break them down, offers another source of healthy fats.

Grains

While many parents find that feeding their children pretzels or Cheerios is an easy option, it's not necessarily the best choice. Consuming refined or wheat-based grains can lead to an imbalanced microflora and inflammation that disrupts the lining of the gastrointestinal tract. Many children have devastating digestive problems, allergies, ADD/ADHD and other issues when consuming wheat based and refined grains. When children stop consuming them, many of their physical and mental symptoms improve.[6]

Water

Drinking clean and sufficient amounts of water is important as children develop to ensure adequate hydration and optimal kidney, brain, cardiovascular, digestive and general cellular function. Hydration requirements change based on your child's age.

Know How Much Water to Give Your Child

For the first six months, breastmilk has sufficient amounts of water in it to meet a baby's hydration needs. From 6–12 months, anywhere from 2–4 ounces of water serves to introduce a new beverage to the babies's palate, helps them drink out of a sippy cup and helps them make the transition from a liquid diet to solid foods. As more solid foods are introduced, more water may be necessary, especially if they are constipated or if the weather is very hot.[7]

As a general rule of thumb, naturopathic doctors will consider half a person's body weight in ounces an adequate amount of water to drink. If a child has pale yellow urine, it generally indicates adequate hydration.

Breastfeeding

The primary source of food for all humans is breastmilk. It is specifically created for newborn infants and babies to meet the needs of their developing bodies. It is full of nutrients such as vitamins, minerals, proteins, carbohydrates, fats, antioxidants, enzymes, probiotics and antibodies that babies need to grow.[8] The longer a child receives breastmilk, the longer protection is available to that child. Studies show that with longer duration of breastfeeding, the stronger their overall immune function is.[9]

Not only does breast milk protect from acute infections, such as ear and respiratory infections, and diarrhea during the early months of life, it supports healthy immune, brain and gastrointestinal development.[10, 11] It also provides long term health support many years into the future to minimize the risk of developing chronic illnesses like allergies, asthma, gastroenteritis and autoimmune diseases.[12, 13, 14]

In addition to the physical support a child receives from breastfeeding, there is also skin-to-skin contact which provides comfort to an infant. The bonding that happens between a mother and child through breastfeeding increases a child's level of confidence and trust in the world. Breastfeeding helps to create a more emotionally balanced child.[15]

The current standard medical recommendation for breastfeeding is currently six months.[16] However, newer research is indicating that prematurely stopping breastfeeding can increase risk for developing autoimmune diseases.[17] This indicates that there is a need for children to breastfeed for longer periods of time. In other countries, mothers breastfeed children for years since these benefits are well understood by new mothers, their families and health providers.[18]

Seeing the benefits that a child receives from breastmilk, it is critically important to provide breastmilk to a child for as long as possible. If, for example, a mother is only able to breastfeed for two weeks because she needs to return to work, then two weeks of breastmilk is better than no breastmilk at all. If she can only breastfeed once a day, that is acceptable as well. Any amount of breastmilk (either through breastfeeding or bottle-feeding) is preferable over not providing it for the overall health of a growing child.

Exercise

Daily exercise is as important to children as fresh air. Increased heart rate and breathing caused by fast walking, running or jumping and increased sweating keep the heart strong, purify the lungs and pump the lymphatic system. This leads to development of a resistant cardiovascular network, optimal lung function and an effective detoxification system. Immunity is also indirectly enhanced because of the elimination of toxins and effective blood circulation that oxygenates numerous body organs.

Get Children to Play

Encouraging your child to engage in physical activity they enjoy—swimming, running around with friends, bicycling, jumping on a trampoline or competing in team sports—will meet the requirements of regular exercise. Also, if they spend time outdoors they'll have the added benefit of sun exposure enhancing their own production of vitamin D.

Teach Them Yoga

Yoga is often described as an "exercise routine" that a person incorporates into their current lifestyle. However, yoga, an ancient sanskrit word, is perhaps better understood through one of its many translations: to

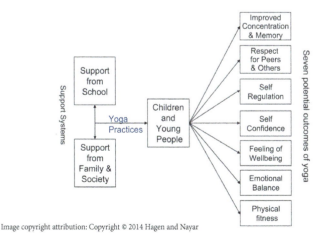

Image copyright attribution: Copyright © 2014 Hagen and Nayar

unite, as in uniting the mind, body and spirit. Yoga does include physical exercise but it also is about life balance: training one's mind, body and breath, as well as connecting to a sense of spirituality.

Yoga combines physical exercises or postures (*asanas*) that build strength, flexibility and confidence with breathing (*pranayama*) which calms and refresh the body and mind. What is really exciting is that yoga has been shown to improve both physical and mental health in school-age children (ages 6–12)[19]. For the purposes of this book, it has specifically been shown to modulate and improve immune function.[20] How exactly practicing yoga does this is being researched, but it is believed that the stress hormones are regulated, thereby decreasing the negative effects of stress hormones on the immune system.

Many gyms, community centers, local yoga studios and YMCAs offer yoga classes. If your child enjoys learning on their own, consider a yoga video or online course. One of the best things about yoga is that children can practice alone, with a friend or with a group. Some specific yoga poses that are great for your child include: child pose, perfect pose, lotus pose and forward bend pose.

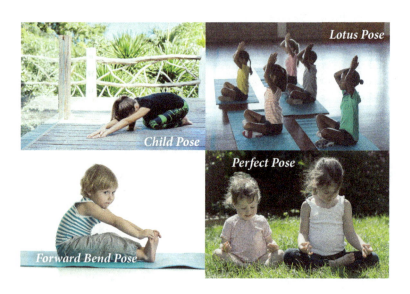

Lotus Pose

Child Pose

Perfect Pose

Forward Bend Pose

Exposure to Microorganisms

If you watch television or look at magazine ads, you will see babies and young children crawling and playing on sparkling clean floors. While it may seem desirable to have small children playing on clean surfaces, the immunological reality is quite different. With decreased exposure to germs (from the use of antibacterial soaps, sprays and cleaning supplies), children's immune system's fail to be exposed to sufficient amounts of microorganisms and they will be unable to mount an immune response when it is required. This is seen in the rising rates of children with allergies, autoimmune conditions and gut disorders.[21] Bacteria-poor indoor environments breed children with increased cases of asthma and allergies, which are signs of immune dysfunction.

Playing in the Dirt

Researchers have come to recognize *that literally playing in the dirt* is beneficial to a child's developing immune system because of increased exposure to various microorganisms. When looking at immunological regulation and exposure to worms, there is inhibition of different T helper (Th) cells depending on the type of immunological response being made. Inflammatory diseases like asthma and Crohn's disease were decreased because of inhibition of Th17[22] (a T helper cell involved in the development of autoimmune diseases[23]).

With more bacteria in a child's body, there is enhancement of digestive health, decreases in allergies, and improved mood. The essential microorganisms found in dirt are soil-based organisms. They are hearty enough to survive digestive juices and can be found in a person's body up to one year later after a single exposure.[24]

Get a Pet

Although dogs may not fit every family's structure, studies now find that families with pets support a stronger immune response.[25] Dogs bring microbes into the home via their paws, snout and fur. They offer a wide range of exposure to microbes that children spending a majority of time indoors don't have, and introduce as many as fifty-six different bacterial species into the home.[26] A study comparing traditional farm-raised Amish children (who played with farm animals) to children growing up in industrialized farming communities (who did *not* play with farm animals) showed that the Amish children had 4–6 times less of an allergic response, despite having six times as much house dust in their surroundings.[27] Although most children won't have exposure to farm animals, indoor pets are the next best transporter of necessary microbes.

Stress-Free Zone:
The Importance of Mental and Emotional Health

Stress affects the development of a child's nervous, digestive and immune system. Their nervous and digestive systems must be able to go into rest and digest mode for optimal immune functioning. It's critical to maintain a stress-free zone for the normal and optimal growth and development of a child.

Children today live in a very different world than children from previous generations. The air is polluted, the water has chemicals and is depleted of minerals, the food is also full of chemicals, preservatives, hormones, food coloring and, oftentimes, lacks nutrients because of low nutrient content within the soil. Physically, many children are stressed because of lack of nutrients and high amounts of toxins in the environment. Emotional stress also affects children. They can have their own stressors and can also feel the nervousness and tension their parents are experiencing from work, financial or family stress.

What Does a Stress-Free Zone Look Like?

Children thrive when they feel safe and at peace in their environment. They are very receptive to non-verbal forms of meditation. Calming music in the background can be supportive to their neurological development, as seen with classical music, ambient noise or humming.[28, 29] Additionally, other types of meditation work well for young children. Guided visualization meditations work well to relax children by giving them an image, scene or item to focus on. Studies have shown improvements in resilience to stress and cognitive performance with various meditation techniques.[30] Different types of meditation practices are being used and finding one that works well for a child can make the difference between a child that is well adjusted psychologically and socially or not.

1 Jung C, JP Hugot, and F Barreau. 2010. "Peyer's Patches: The Immune Sensors of the Intestine". *International Journal of Inflammation*. 2010.

2 Belkaid Y, and TW Hand. 2014. "Role of the microbiota in immunity and inflammation". *Cell*. 157 (1): 121-41.

3 Grasa L, L Abecia, R Forcén, M Castro, de Jalón JA, E Latorre, AI Alcalde, and MD Murillo. 2015. "Antibiotic-Induced Depletion of Murine Microbiota Induces Mild Inflammation and Changes in Toll-Like Receptor Patterns and Intestinal Motility". *Microbial Ecology*. 70 (3): 835-48.

4 Langdon, Amy, Crook, Nathan, and Dantas, Gautam. 2016. *The effects of antibiotics on the microbiome throughout development and alternative approaches for therapeutic modulation*. BioMed Central Ltd.

5 Murray, Michael T., and Joseph E. Pizzorno. 2014. The encyclopedia of natural medicine.

6 Ghalichi F, J Ghaemmaghami, A Malek, and A Ostadrahimi. 2016. "Effect of gluten free diet on gastrointestinal and behavioral indices for children with autism spectrum disorders: a randomized clinical trial". *World Journal of Pediatrics* : WJP. 12 (4): 436-442.

7 Shu, Jennifer. "How much water do babies need to drink?" CNN. http://www.cnn.com/2009/HEALTH/expert.q.a/07/20/babies.water.drink.shu/index.html

8 Cerini, C., and G. M. Aldrovandi. 2013. "Breast milk: proactive immunomodulation and mucosal protection against viruses and other pathogens". *FUTURE VIROLOGY*. 8 (11): 1127-1134.

9 Hanson, Lars A. 1998. "Breastfeeding Provides Passive and Likely Long-Lasting Active Immunity". *Annals of Allergy, Asthma & Immunology*. 81 (6): 523-537.

10 Ibid

11 Brown University. "Breastfeeding benefits babies' brains." Brown.edu https://news.brown.edu/articles/2013/06/breastfeeding (accessed September 28, 2017)

12 Hanson, Lars A. 1998. "Breastfeeding Provides Passive and Likely Long-Lasting Active Immunity". *Annals of Allergy, Asthma & Immunology*. 81 (6): 523-537.

13 Cerini, C., and G. M. Aldrovandi. 2013. "Breast milk: proactive immunomodulation and mucosal protection against viruses and other pathogens". *FUTURE VIROLOGY*. 8 (11): 1127-1134.

14 Office of Women's Health, U.S. Department of Health and Human Services. "Making the decision to breastfeed." Womenshealth.gov. https://www.womenshealth.gov/breastfeeding/making-decision-breastfeed (accessed September 28, 2017)

15 Narvaez, Darcia. "The Tremendous Benefits of Doing What is Normal: Breastfeeding." Psychology Today. https://www.psychologytoday.com/blog/

moral-landscapes/201108/the-tremendous-benefits-doing-what-is-normal-breastfeeding (accessed September 28, 2017)

16 WebMD. "Breastfeeding Overview." WebMD.com https://www.webmd.com/ parenting/baby/nursing-basics#2 (accessed September 28, 2017))

17 Jackson KM, and AM Nazar. 2006. "Breastfeeding, the immune response, and long-term health". *The Journal of the American Osteopathic Association.* 106 (4): 203-7.

18 Colette Young, Priscilla. "Beyond Toddlerhood: The Breastfeeding Relationship Continues." The Natural Child Project. http://www.naturalchild. org/guest/priscilla_colletto.html (accessed September 28, 2017)

19 Hagen I., and Nayar U.S. 2014. "Yoga for children and young people's mental health and well-being: Research review and reflections on the mental health potentials of yoga". *Frontiers in Psychiatry.* 5 (APR).

20 Gopal A., Mondal S., Gandhi A., Arora S., and Bhattacharjee J. 2011. "Effect of integrated yoga practices on immune responses in examination stress-A preliminary study". *International Journal of Yoga.* 4 (1): 26-32.).

21 Brody, Jane. "Babies Know: A Little Dirt Is Good For You." The New York Times. http://www.nytimes.com/2009/01/27/health/27brod.html?_ r=1&adxnnl=1&adxnnlx=1426907280-1gdxnMvnA3pCD5Qul+96sw (accessed August 24, 2017)

22 Ibid

23 Ouyang, Wenjun, Jay K. Kolls, and Yan Zheng. 2008. "The Biological Functions of T Helper 17 Cell Effector Cytokines in Inflammation". Immunity. 28 (4): 454-467.

24 Bittner AC, RM Croffut, MC Stranahan, and TN Yokelson. 2007. "Prescript-assist probiotic-prebiotic treatment for irritable bowel syndrome: an open-label, partially controlled, 1-year extension of a previously published controlled clinical trial". *Clinical Therapeutics.* 29 (6): 1153-60.

25 Schiffman, Richard. "Are Pets The New Probiotic?" The New York Times https://www.nytimes.com/2017/06/06/well/family/are-pets-the-new-probiotic.html (accessed August 24, 2017).

26 Ibid .

27 Stein, Michelle M., Cara L. Hrusch, Justyna Gozdz, Catherine Igartua, Vadim Pivniouk, Sean E. Murray, Julie G. Ledford, et al. 2016. "Innate Immunity and Asthma Risk in Amish and Hutterite Farm Children". *New England Journal of Medicine.* 375 (5): 411-421.

28 Campbell, Don G. 2009. *The Mozart effect for children: awakening your child's mind, health, and creativity with music.* Pymble, NSW: HarperCollins e-books.

29 Gaynor, Mitchell L. 2002. *The healing power of sound: recovery from life-threatening illness using sound, voice, and music.* Boston: Shambhala.

30 Zenner C, S Herrnleben-Kurz, and H Walach. 2014. "Mindfulness-based interventions in schools-a systematic review and meta-analysis". *Frontiers in Psychology*. 5.

PART II:
Naturopathic Modalities (Therapies)

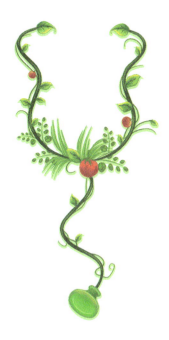

This part of the book will introduce parents and caregivers to different types of therapies that are both natural and safe to use with children. Many can be done at home, while others may need to be performed by a trained professional. This section serves as an introduction to each therapy and focuses on the way these therapies work to support health and recovery from illness. The Apothecary section contains more detailed information on how to use these particular therapies either at home or by a professional.

Chapter 3:
The Tools

Botanical Medicine

Humans have co-evolved with plants in a way to help each other mutually. Humans have protected and cultivated specific plants for millennia because they have identified them as allies. Similarly, plants have shared their healing attributes with humans while using those same phytochemicals to heal themselves from harsh environments like flooding, heat waves, cold winters, or insect invasion.

Botanical medicine is the centuries-old method of using herbs and plants to heal. This is a practice that is used around the world, whether or not pharmaceutical agents are available. Humans consume herbs in the form of teas, tinctures, glycerites, salves, poultices, baths, essential oils, syrups, tablets or capsules. Herbs can be used for children of all ages from newborn onward. Many herbal formulas are available, and you'll see our discussion of them throughout the book. Here are descriptions of each so you know the differences between them:

- ◆ Bath: Herbal baths can include any combination of herbs. Place herbs inside a muslin bag or cheesecloth and drop it into warm bath or hold it under hot water stream.

- ◆ Capsules: Powdered herb or herbs placed into a capsule and swallowed. These can be used for numerous health concerns.

- ◆ Essential oils: Oil extracts from numerous plants are available for a variety of health concerns including physical immune enhancement, emotional balancing and physical and mental relaxation.

- ◆ Glycerite: A liquid preparation of an herb made using vegetable glycerin to extract the medicinal constituents of the plant. It tastes sweet which makes it more palatable for children.

- ◆ Salve: A semi-solid herbal preparation usually made with beeswax, olive oil (or some other type of carrier oil), dried herbs and essential oils (if desired). Salves are used topically for burns, wounds, rashes, boils or other skin conditions.

- Syrup: A viscous herbal preparation usually made with honey and varying herbs. It is used to soothe a sore throat.

- Tablets: Single herbs or a combination of herbs blended together and either chewed or swallowed. These are generally used for sore throats or for children who don't like taking liquid herbs.

- Tea: Adding hot water to a dried herb, allowing it to steep for a few minutes, removing the herbs and drinking it once it has cooled down. Teas can be used for colds, coughs, relaxation, sleep problems, urinary complaints and more.

- Tincture: A liquid preparation of an herb through an alcohol or alcohol and water extraction process. It is usually made in a 1:5 ratio with one part of herb being diluted in five parts of water. The dosage is measured in drops. They can be used for many conditions including coughs, colds, fevers, flus or any time immune activation is desired.

Essential Oils[1]

For treating infections, essential oils are a vital part of a home medicine chest. In the late 1800s, scientists studying essential oils discovered they were very effective in addressing a wide variety of infectious diseases. Much of this research, however, was abandoned after the discovery of antibiotics. As the age of miracle drugs draws near (researchers have not discovered a new class of antibiotics since the 1970s), and more and more microbes are developing resistance to antibiotics, researchers are once again turning to essential oils as a powerful way of addressing bacterial, viral and fungal infections.[2] In addition to treating infections, essentials oils also help soothe the symptoms associated with those illnesses.

Essential oils comprise about 1–2% of most plants. Because they are potent (and potentially damaging) volatile oils, plants wall them off in vacuoles and release them only when needed: to ward off insect invasion, heal a bruise or break, or combat disease.

When essential oils are used, that plant's healing intelligence is "borrowed". Numerous studies confirm that essential oils can affect your moods, reduce pain levels, heal wounds, fight infections and more.[3, 4]

Safety First

You can use essential oils in many safe and effective ways, but we don't recommend ingesting them. Some essential oil companies claim you can ingest their essential oils because they are "pure." Just because something is pure does not mean it is safe to ingest. Gasoline, for example, is very pure, but we would NOT recommend ingesting it.

For humans, one drop of an essential oil is roughly equivalent to drinking 30 cups of tea in terms of active ingredients. Because essential oils are so potent, taking essential oils by mouth can overstimulate phase I and II liver detoxification pathways and lead to liver damage. Instead, rely on skin applications and inhalation of essential oils. Research shows inhaling essential oils or applying them to the skin causes a rapid rise of the active constituents in the bloodstream within seconds of application.[5, 6, 7]

> **Caution: Babies and young children have very thin and sensitive skin. Undiluted essential oils can overstimulate them and cause skin reactions, such as rashes or spasmodic coughing. Use essential oils mixed with a carrier oil, almond, coconut or olive work well, when using essential oils with babies and young children.**

Organic, Authentic Essential Oils

Choose authentic essential oils. Many of the large essential oil companies "broker" essential oils, meaning they contract chemical companies to create oils that include only a fraction of all of the active constituents in an essential oil. These brokered oils do not have the same therapeutic effect as an *authentic* essential oil.

Some essential oil companies substitute related species for the plant listed on the bottle. Although these oils smell similar, they do not have the same therapeutic effect. *Lavandin*, for example, is often sold as "lavender," but is a different genus than true lavender, *Lavandula angustifolia*. Only buy essential oils that list the plant genus and species on the bottle.

Also, make sure you are choosing organic essential oils. Pesticides are very similar in molecular size to essential oils, and they will travel along with the essential oil in the distillation process. If you are uncertain about whether the oils you are using are organic, you can ask the manufacturer to provide you with a gas chromatography report. This report verifies the characteristic "fingerprint" of constituents for that particular oil, and reveals whether the oil has been contaminated with pesticides or adulterated with other products.

Less is More

Increasing the concentration of an essential oil may actually *decrease* its effectiveness. Often a 1–2% dilution is enough![8, 9]

Use Small Amounts Frequently

Using diluted preparations of essential oils several times during the day gives you the greatest benefit. As an example, people given lavender essential oil on a cotton ball to inhale *once* a day for twenty minutes for two days after open-heart surgery had no reduction in anxiety.[10] Another group inhaling lavender essential oil *twice* daily for twenty minutes had a significant reduction in anxiety,[11] while people in a longer-term (fifteen days) study with twice daily inhalation had less anxiety as well as improvements in sleep and depression.[12]

The bottom line: use dilute preparations of essential oils several times a day for maximum benefit.

Essential Oils for Young Children and Babies

Only a handful of essential oils are safe for babies and young children (applied in any form):

Babies (birth-18 months): Dosage 1/6 adult dosage

- ♦ Lavender

- ♦ Roman chamomile

- ♦ Rose

Toddlers (18 months-4 years): Dosage ¼ adult dosage

- ♦ All of the oils listed for babies plus

- ♦ *Eucalyptus radiata* (not the more common *Eucalyptus globulus,* which is a stronger, more stimulating essential oil)

     ◆ Mandarin Tangerine

     ◆ Tea Tree

5-12 year olds: Dosage ½ adult dosage

     ◆ All of the oils listed for babies and toddlers plus

     ◆ Citruses (e.g. grapefruit, orange)

     ◆ Spearmint

Methods for Using Essential Oils

METHOD 1: Inhalation

When you breathe in essential oils, they penetrate the cells lining the lungs and cross immediately into the bloodstream. As you inhale, essential oils also cross the blood-brain barrier and directly influence the brain.[13]

You can explore three methods for inhaling essential oils: inhaler, diffuser and mister.

Inhaler

Inhalers are a wonderfully convenient way to use essential oils. You can carry one in your pocket or purse or store next to your bedside. Using an inhaler targets delivery so not everyone in the room (or on the plane or train) is exposed to the essential oils.

You can buy "blank" inhalers in most health-food stores or from online sources.

You can benefit from essential oils even if you have no sense of smell. If you can smell,[14] you will be more likely to use the inhaler if you enjoy the scent. Research shows those who used the inhaler more frequently had greater benefit.[15]

   To use an essential oil inhaler:

     ◆ Use a total of 8–10 drops of an individual essential oil or an essential oil blend

     ◆ Saturate the cotton wick with 8–10 drops of essential oil

- Place the wick inside the tube

- Insert the cap at the end of the tube

- Screw the tube into the outer casing

- "Recharge" the wick every 2–3 months by removing the cap and saturating the wick with another 8–10 drops of essential oil. Always recharge with the same essential oils.

Mister

Even at levels too low to consciously smell, essential oils diffused into a room can improve mood, increase concentration and reduce bacteria and viruses in the air.[16]

It's best to choose glass spray bottles to contain your mists, as essential oils will degrade plastic over time, and to opt for dark blue or amber glass to help prevent light from damaging your blends. Glass spray bottles can be surprisingly difficult to find in stores, but you can find them from many online sources.

To use an essential oil mister:

- Fill an 8 ounce mister with water

- Add 1–2 tablespoons of alcohol (vodka or pure-grain alcohol). Alcohol helps disperse the essential oil in water.

- For a 1% concentration, add 48 drops of a single essential oil or a blend. For a 2% concentration, add 96 drops.

- Shake the bottle before misting. Even if you can no longer smell the essential oils after 15–20 minutes, their therapeutic effect will continue. Repeat the misting 3–4 times a day.

Diffuser

You can diffuse essential oils in a variety of ways. Heating essential oils oxidizes them and creates caustic substances that damage the lungs and other tissues.[17] Please use non-heat methods to diffuse the oils.

Examples of safe diffusers:

+ Terra cotta figures impregnated with essential oils

+ A few drops of essential oil on a cotton ball or Kleenex

+ Cold mist diffusers

Suggested Essential Oils for Inhalation

These essential oils can be used with any of the inhalation delivery methods: inhalers, misters or diffusers.

+ Anxiety: lavender,[18] lemongrass,[19] ylang ylang[20, 21]

+ Increased concentration: rosemary,[22, 23] basil, peppermint

+ Sleep: lavender,[24] lemon balm, ylang ylang

+ Bronchodilation: eucalyptus

+ Anti-inflammatory for nasal passages: peppermint[25]

+ Antibacterial: thyme, tea tree, eucalyptus; pine and other conifers; lemon and other citrus family members.[26, 27, 28] (One effective combination is: Siberian fir and grapefruit.)

METHOD 2: Topical Application

Vegetable oil with essential oil

Make a 1% or 2% dilution. Choose a pure, organic carrier vegetable oil such as almond, avocado, safflower, sunflower, coconut or olive oil.

+ To make a 1% dilution: Add one drop of essential oil to a teaspoon of pure, organic vegetable oil OR three drops of essential oil to a tablespoon of pure, organic vegetable oil.

+ To make a 2% dilution: Add two drops of essential oil to a teaspoon of pure, organic vegetable oil OR six drops of essential oil to a tablespoon of pure, organic vegetable oil.

+ For children under six years old, dilute one drop of an essential oil in two tablespoons of pure, organic vegetable oil.

Rub the diluted essential oil into the affected area (e.g. the chest for a cough, the forehead and temples for a headache). **Always avoid the eyes and ear canals when you apply essential oils.**

Salve or Lip Balm

This recipe can be used either for salve or lip balm, although you may need to adjust the amount of beeswax slightly depending on how firm or soft you want the salve or lip balm to be.

- In a double boiler (or a heat-proof bowl over a pot of water), gently melt 2 ounce of beeswax over low heat

- Add 1 cup of pure, organic vegetable oil such as almond, avocado, safflower, coconut, olive or sunflower.

- Test the thickness of the salve or lip balm by putting a teaspoon of the oil-beeswax combination in the freezer

- If you want a softer consistency, add another teaspoon or two of oil and retest

- If you want a firmer consistency, add a small amount of beeswax and retest

- When you have the consistency you want, remove from heat, then stir in either a single essential oil or a combination for a total of 48–96 drops (1–2% concentration)

- Quickly pour into shallow glass or metal jars for salves; pour into small jars or tubes for lip balm

- Allow to cool completely before putting on the lids

- Keep the lid on when the salve or lip balm is not in use so that essential oils do not evaporate. Always label herbal salves and lip balms.

Suggested Essential Oils for Topical Use

These essential oils make good therapeutic blends for salves and lip balms.

- Soothing and healing the skin: lavender, helichrysum, St. John's wort, rosemary verbenone, rose, German chamomile

♦ Chest congestion: pine, Siberian fir, pinon pine, eucalyptus (use *Eucalyptus radiata* for children).

Caution: When making topical herb products, remember to use only pure, natural ingredients, as they will absorb deeply into the skin. Avoid adding essential oils to products that contain mineral oil or other petroleum products, parabens and/or sodium laureth or lauryl sulfate. Current research demonstrates essential oils can enhance the absorption of many potent drugs and chemicals.[29]

If you want to take essential oils internally, work with a healthcare provider with advanced training. For example, in France, a physician will send orders to a compounding pharmacy to make internal (oral, rectal or vaginal) essential oil prescriptions. Usually physicians prescribe essential oils for internal use for a maximum of fourteen days.

Certifications to look for when choosing a healthcare provider to help you with essential oils are:

♦ National certification: National Association for Holistic Aromatherapy (NAHA) Certified Clinical Aromatherapist®

♦ International certification: Alliance of International Aromatherapists (AIA)

Homeopathy

Homeopathy is a system of medicine that is over 200 years old and may be one of the safest and most effective therapies in medicine. The "medicines" used in homeopathy are commonly referred to as "remedies". These remedies are highly diluted substances that contain little to no molecules of the substance they are made from, but they do contain the information of the original substance. It is believed that this information stimulates the innate healing ability of the body, restoring balance and thereby allowing the symptoms of illness to resolve.

Homeopathic remedies come in a variety of strengths. The common strengths available in most health food stores are 6C and 30C, but other strengths such as 200C are available online and from holistic doctors such as naturopathic and homeopathic doctors. Homeopathic remedies are easy and affordable to obtain. No prescription is needed for a homeopathic remedy, and the typical cost is around $10.00 for 80–100 pellets.

Most remedies come as little white pellets to which a homeopathic medicine has been applied. They are about the size of a poppy seed (although some brands make pellets that are slightly larger), and the remedy is usually chewed or placed under the tongue. For very young children, the pellets can be crushed and mixed with water. Typically, you use one remedy at a time, but there are some combination products available that contain two or more homeopathic medicines.

Homeopathic treatment is good for first aid, acute and chronic illness, and is especially effective for treating many of the childhood illnesses discussed in the Conditions section. Treatment using homeopathy can be very rewarding, since it is inexpensive and children tend to respond quickly. A correctly chosen remedy can work gently and efficiently to relieve discomfort and help the body heal itself without toxicity or side effects. However, there are a few important rules to follow to get the best results with homeopathy.

First, you need to make a list of all your child's symptoms, as those will lead you to the best remedy. The key to the symptoms is all in the details. Here are two lists of symptoms. The first list has very general symptoms, while the symptoms on the second list are more specific. The specific list of symptoms will help you choose the best remedy. It is very important to note that. Anything that is different from normal can be important, including their mental or emotional state.

General

- complains they are cold

- says their throat hurts

- fussy, clearly does not feel well

- won't eat

- has a stuffy nose

Specific

- your child's hands and feet feel cold (to the child) but when you feel their hands and feet, they feel warmer than usual

◆ their throat hurts on the left side, especially when they are trying to swallow food and feels better when they drink something, especially something hot

◆ they are fussy and want to be held by you, constantly

◆ they do not want to be left alone

◆ when prompted about eating anything they want at all they ask for a spoon of peanut butter

◆ their nose is stuffy on the left, but the right side seems clear

◆ when they blow their nose, the mucus is thick and greenish-yellow

To get the most specific symptoms, you will have to both observe and ask your child questions. How you ask the question can be very important, as children usually seek to please their caregiver. Of course, if your child is not old enough to talk, this becomes all about your power of observation. Here are a couple of good and not so good questions:

◆ Good: Show me where your throat hurts.

◆ Not so good: Does your throat hurt here?

◆ Good: Take a drink of this (something cold) and then this (something warm). Which one makes it feel better?

◆ Not so good: Does something cold to drink make it feel better?

After you have ascertained your child's symptoms, you must choose the most correct remedy. This is one of the most important concepts in homeopathy. How do you know which is the most correct remedy? Quite simply, it is the remedy whose listed symptoms most closely match the illness symptoms.

As an example of this we will use the homeopathic remedy, Belladonna (Bell.). For a child with a fever for whom Belladonna could be very helpful you would likely see the following symptoms: a rapidly developing fever, very hot skin, flushed face, pounding or throbbing pains in the head (or other parts of the body), extreme restlessness, dilated pupils and little to no perspiration. If these are the symptoms that your child has, it is likely Belladonna would help.

If the fever had slowly crept up over a few days, the child was kind of chilly, very sweaty, listless (not restless), then Belladonna would probably not help. So, the point here is that there is not a single remedy for a fever, but rather a particular remedy for a particular fever. This second example of a fever would need a completely different remedy.

Finally, the dosing of the homeopathic remedy can be very important. In this book, we only suggest 30C strengths. But in fact there are many additional strengths, such as 200C, 1M and higher. Many homeopathic doctors will provide a small kit that contains remedies in both the 30C and 200C strengths. Dosing can be different from one child to the next. In one child, a single dose of 30C may be all that is needed to set things right whereas in another child, 8–10 doses of 30C may be needed. There is no way to predict what your child will need, but it is pretty easy to figure out once you have given the first dose.

Dose once and observe. The symptoms may get slightly worse right after dosing and then improvement should be seen. As long as your child is improving, do not redose. When your child stops improving or when the symptoms seem like they are getting worse, redose. If there is no improvement after the first dose, try a second dose. If there is no change at all in the symptoms, it is either the wrong dosage or the wrong remedy.

If there is improvement after every dose of a remedy but improvement stops and symptoms have NOT continued to change, then it is likely your child needs a higher strength of the remedy. Try the 200C instead of the 30C. If the symptoms HAVE changed, they may need a different remedy. Here are some examples to help clarify this:

Example 1: Your child needs the same remedy at higher strength

Symptoms: rapidly developing fever, very hot, pounding or throbbing pains in the head (or other parts of the body), extreme restlessness, dilated pupils and little to no perspiration. Bell 30C given. Symptoms start improving in that fever is less, throbbing pains less, restlessness decreases. That lasts for a couple of hours. Then the fever starts to rise again, they feel hot, hands and feet are cold, throbbing pain comes back, restlessness returns. You would redose Bell 30C. The symptoms improve again. This happens 5 times. After the 5th dose there is no improvement and no difference in the symptoms. They need a higher strength, Bell 200C.

Example 2: Your child needs a different remedy

Same example as above, except after the 5th dose they seem to have different symptoms. Instead of feeling hot they are now very cold, they have a sharp pain at the top of their head (different kind of pain), they want to be all covered up and are worse when uncovered, air blowing on them makes them very irritable and sounds are bothering them. These are different symptoms and Bell does not cover symptoms like these. They need a different remedy, probably Nux vomica. You would start the new remedy at the 30C strength.

Children will often feel better before they are better. Even if all the symptoms are gone, allow for rest and recovery, otherwise known as convalescence.

How to Use Homeopathic Remedies for the Conditions in This Book

Along with each illness described in The Conditions section, we describe several possible homeopathic remedies. Most of the conditions have a remedy listed at the beginning as part of the "homeopathic prophylactic protocol." This is a remedy that is used by homeopathic doctors in lieu of the vaccination for that illness. With a couple of exceptions, which are noted within any given condition, the homeopathic prophylactic protocol remedy is not typically used to treat the illness once present. The remaining remedies listed in the homeopathy part of each condition are common remedies to consider to treat the illness. It is important to note that these are the most common remedies used but they may not be the only remedies to consider. The remedies are listed by their full name followed by the common abbreviation in parentheses.

The symptoms that any given homeopathic remedy can be used to treat have been compiled into a vast collection of information called the *Homeopathic Materia Medica*. There are many different materia medicas to choose from. In this book, we have used several different materia medicas and selected symptoms that are specific to each condition to help you choose the best possible remedy. Your child does not need to have all of the symptoms listed within a remedy (and often they will not). You do want to be sure that the remedy you choose has most, if not all, of the symptoms of your child.

It may be a little challenging at first to read the description of each remedy. But keep at it and you will get the hang of it in no time at all. Just keep in mind, these are just a list of possible symptoms your child may have. You do not have to worry about choosing the wrong remedy; you are not hurting your child. They simply won't improve as they would with the correctly chosen remedy. Try again! There is no mistaking a positive homeopathic response and once you see it you will know what you are looking for. Helpful homeopathy books to have on hand at home are listed in the Resources section.

Hydrotherapy

Hydrotherapy uses water as a method of healing. Although considered an old world therapy, it is commonly used today in spas around the world in the form of jacuzzis and steam rooms. A spa setting is meant for relaxation and stress release but when used therapeutically for children it is much more than simply relaxation.

In *Lectures on Naturopathic Hydrotherapy*, the authors discuss various methods of hydrotherapy used for children and adults to stimulate immune function, increase blood circulation and amplify natural detoxification. Their discussion covers treatments like:

- ◆ Alternating sheet wraps: alternating hot and cold sheets to increase circulation of oxygen and immune cells

- ◆ Baths: to support a fever

- ◆ Cooling towels: to relieve a child with a fever

- ◆ Steam inhalation: placing face over warm steam to open up the sinuses

- ◆ Wet socks: putting cold wet cotton socks on with a pair of wool socks over top to increase immune function

It can safely be used with babies (think of taking a baby with a congested nose into a bathroom with a hot shower running) or children (use of wet socks to stimulate immune function). Some hydrotherapy treatments are better suited for specific conditions. The most appropriate type of hydrotherapy treatment will be discussed within the context of specific conditions.

Mind-Body Connection

Chronic stress has led to the development of many illnesses.[30] This shows the strong connection the mind has on the body. Children feel their parents' stress and react to what they are feeling. It can show up as long bouts of crying, not wanting to go to bed or temper tantrums. Emotional outbursts, which are experienced as physical stress, deplete children's immune function. Even for children that aren't yet verbal, the way a parent or caregiver handles a situation will be felt by the child and will provide information about how to face conflict and stress in life.

A study published in the *Journal of Immunology*[31] showed that children who experienced serious life events, stress or worry from parents and lack of social support had higher levels of cortisol and a predisposition to develop higher blood sugar levels which could lead to type I diabetes. This makes sense in psychoneuroimmunological terms, considering how the mind can affect either resistance to or support for health.[32] Interestingly, new research shows how our perspective on stress can either positively or negatively affect our health. If stress is perceived as a challenge or something to overcome, the physical body thrives. If it is viewed as a detriment, the body starts to underfunction and becomes sick. This is an important difference to keep in mind since, as parents or caregivers, you have the power to create a positive or negative experience for your child or children in your life.

Ultimately, when parents create a peaceful, safe and harmonious environment for children, development ensues naturally and normally.[33] Maintaining a conflict-free home is not always possible, but using conflict as a teaching opportunity about hardiness can make a considerable difference in the health of your child.

Nutrition

As discussed previously, a proper diet is key to creating and restoring health. Creating the optimal nutritional status within your child's body before they become ill is the best strategy! This gives your child's body what it needs in order to mount an immune response and recover from illness more quickly.

For example, consider streptococcus bacteria, which is widespread among the human population. However, not everyone gets sick with "strep throat." Why is that? Research has clearly shown that the condition of health within a person who is exposed to pathogens plays a huge role in whether or not they get sick, how sick they become and how quickly they recover.[34] Nutritional therapies can also be used as a treatment. For example, a hot, rich broth-based soup can encourage the immune system to work better.

Physical Medicine

Physical medicine includes a wide range of therapies used by practitioners such as naturopathic doctors, chiropractic doctors, acupuncturists, osteopathic doctors and physical therapists. Some practitioners use physical medicine to restore proper structure to the body which then encourages proper function within the body. Others employ physical medicine therapies, to stimulate healing processes within the body. For example, lymphatic massage encourages the circulation of lymph and can help immune function by moving metabolic by-products from the tissues into the nodes, where they can be neutralized. Other examples of physical medicine techniques that can be beneficial include skeletal realignment, muscle massage, dry skin brushing, abdominal massage and craniosacral realignment.

Many of these therapies, such as muscle massage, lymphatic massage and dry skin brushing, can be done at home to help encourage health and healing. Other therapies, such as skeletal realignment, are best done by someone with specialized training. Either way, most children, when feeling under the weather, do much better with physical touch—as in the soothing and calming hand of a caring parent, family member or health provider—hence, the old adage "the healing power of touch."

Topical and External Applications

Using topical and external applications is beneficial for much more than treating the skin. You may be familiar with applying a cream to a cut or scrape but there is also powerful medicine to be found for the inner workings of the body through external applications. These types of therapies can include:

♦ Compress (castor oil pack): A cloth soaked in a solution and like a poultice is applied topically that is designed to ease painful joints and muscles, draw out infection or deliver plant medicine through the skin. Another word for compress is fomentation.

♦ Hydrotherapy applications: As discussed in the previous section, applications such as magic socks, medicated heat or cold packs and baths with medicine added to water.

♦ Liniment liquid or semi-liquid preparation (mint chest rub): Used for delivering medicine, often essential oils or herbal medicine, through the skin.

♦ Poultice (e.g. onion poultice, mustard poultice, garlic socks): A warm mass of herbs, or some other plant material applied topically that is designed to ease painful joints and muscles, draw out infection or deliver plant medicine through the skin.

In addition to soothing aching muscles and joints and delivering medicine, topical and external applications can also stimulate healing processes. They can encourage blood flow, relieve the body of heat and help the body eliminate toxins and waste products. *Some general rules to follow are to always check the temperature of the application to be sure it is not too hot or cold, use a timer and do not use anything your child has shown an allergic reaction to previously. For example, if your child has an allergy to onion, never use an onion poultice.*

We have included more detailed information in The Apothecary section for topical applications. We have also listed good books and places to purchase products in the Resources section.

1 Judith Boice ND, LAc, FABNO

2 Yap P.S.X., Yiap B.C., Lim S.H.E., and Ping H.C. 2014. "Essential Oils, a New Horizon in Combating Bacterial Antibiotic Resistance". *Open Microbiology Journal.* 8: 6-14.

3 Edris, Amr E. 2007. "Pharmaceutical and therapeutic Potentials of essential oils and their individual volatile constituents: a review". *Phytotherapy Research.* 21 (4): 308-323.

4 Herz, Rachel S. 2009. "Aromatherapy Facts and Fictions: A Scientific Analysis of Olfactory Effects on Mood, Physiology and Behavior". *International Journal of Neuroscience.* 119 (2): 263-290.

5 Jager, W., Buchbauer, G. et al. 1992. "Percutaneous absorption of lavender oil from a massage oil." *Journal of the Society of Cosmetic Chemists.* 43: 49–54.

6 Valette, C. 1945. "Penetration transcutanee des essences." Comptes Rendues Societe Biologique.

7 Buchbauer, G. 1993. Molecular Interaction. *International Journal of Aromatherapy.* 5 (1): 11-14.

8 Boyd EM, and EP Sheppard. 1968. "The effect of steam inhalation of volatile oils on the output and composition of respiratory tract fluid". *The Journal of Pharmacology and Experimental Therapeutics.* 163 (1): 250-6.

9 Wagner, H and L Sprinkmeyer. 1973. "Uber die pharmakologische Wirkung von Mellissengeist." *Deutsche Apotheker Zeitun* 113 (30): 1159-66.

10 Seifi Z, A Beikmoradi, K Oshvandi, J Poorolajal, M Araghchian, and R Safiaryan. 2014. "The effect of lavender essential oil on anxiety level in patients undergoing coronary artery bypass graft surgery: A double-blinded randomized clinical trial". *Iranian Journal of Nursing and Midwifery Research.* 19 (6): 574-80.

11 Najafi Z., Sharifi K., Tagharrobi Z., Taghadosi M., and Farrokhian A. 2014. "The effects of inhalation aromatherapy on anxiety in patients with myocardial infarction: A randomized clinical trial". *Iranian Red Crescent Medical Journal.* 16 (8).

12 Karadag, E., S. Samancioglu, D. Ozden, and E. Bakir. 2017. "Effects of aromatherapy on sleep quality and anxiety of patients". *NURSING IN CRITICAL CARE.* 22 (2): 105-112.

13 Anthony, CP, and Thibodeau, GA. 1983. Nervous system cells in anatomy and physiology. Mosby, St. Louis

14 Chioca, Lea R., Valqu??ria D.C. Antunes, Marcelo M. Ferro, Estela M. Losso, and Roberto Andreatini. 2013. "Anosmia does not impair the anxiolytic-like effect of lavender essential oil inhalation in mice". *Life Sciences.* 92 (20-21): 971-975.

15 Dyer, Jeannie, Lise Cleary, Maxine Ragsdale-Lowe, Sara McNeill, and Caroline Osland. 2014. "The use of aromasticks at a cancer centre: A

retrospective audit". *Complementary Therapies in Clinical Practice.* 20 (4): 203-206.

16 Naito, Yuko. February 5, 2001. "Just Follow Your Nose, It (Almost) Always Knows." Japan Times.

17 Turek, Claudia, and Florian C. Stintzing. 2013. "Stability of Essential Oils: A Review". *Comprehensive Reviews in Food Science and Food Safety.* 12 (1): 40-53.

18 Karadag, E., S. Samancioglu, D. Ozden, and E. Bakir. 2017. "Effects of aromatherapy on sleep quality and anxiety of patients". *NURSING IN CRITICAL CARE.* 22 (2): 105-112. .

19 Goes TC, FR Ursulino, TH Almeida-Souza, PB Alves, and F Teixeira-Silva. 2015. "Effect of Lemongrass Aroma on Experimental Anxiety in Humans". *Journal of Alternative and Complementary Medicine* (New York, N.Y.). 21 (12): 766-73. .

20 Kim, In-Hee, Kim, Chan, Seong, Kayeon, Hur, Myung-Haeng, Lim, Heon Man, and Lee, Myeong Soo. 2012. Essential Oil Inhalation on Blood Pressure and Salivary Cortisol Levels in Prehypertensive and Hypertensive Subjects. Hindawi Publishing Corporation. http://dx.doi.org/10.1155/2012/984203.

21 Moss, Mark, Steven Hewitt, Lucy Moss, And Keith Wesnes. 2009. "Modulation Of Cognitive Performance And Mood By Aromas Of Peppermint And Ylang-ylang". *International Journal of Neuroscience.* 118 (1): 59-77.

22 Moss, Mark, and Lorraine Oliver. 2012. "Plasma 1,8-cineole correlates with cognitive performance following exposure to rosemary essential oil aroma". *Therapeutic Advances in Psychopharmacology.* 2 (3): 103-113.

23 Hope, Jenny. "Why a whiff of rosemary DOES help you remember: Sniffing the herb can increase memory by 75%." dailymail.co.uk. http://www. dailymail.co.uk/health/article-2306078/Why-whiff-rosemary-does-help-remember.html (accessed Jan 3, 2017).

24 Karadag, E., S. Samancioglu, D. Ozden, and E. Bakir. 2017. "Effects of aromatherapy on sleep quality and anxiety of patients". *NURSING IN CRITICAL CARE.* 22 (2): 105-112.

25 Gao M., Singh A., Macri K., Reynolds C., Singhal V., Biswal S., and Spannhake E.W. 2011. "Antioxidant components of naturally-occurring oils exhibit marked anti-inflammatory activity in epithelial cells of the human upper respiratory system". *Respiratory Research.* 12.

26 Belaiche, P. 1979. "Traité de phytothérapie et d aromathérapie, tome 2: maladies infectieuses." Paris: Maloine S.A.

27 Janssen, A. M., J. J. C. Scheffer, and A. Baerheim Svendsen. 1987. "Antimicrobial Activity of Essential Oils: A 1976-1986 Literature Review. Aspects of the Test Methods". *Planta Med.* 53 (5): 395-398.

28 Price, Shirley, and Len Price. 2015. Aromatherapy for health professionals. Edinburgh [etc.]: Churchill Livingstone. NEW)

29 Herman, Anna, and Andrzej P. Herman. 2015. "Essential oils and their constituents as skin penetration enhancer for transdermal drug delivery: a review". *Journal of Pharmacy and Pharmacology*. 67 (4): 473-485.

30 Salleh, M. R. 2008. "Life Event, Stress and Illness". The Malaysian Journal of Medical Sciences : MJMS, 15(4), 9–18. .

31 Carlsson E., Faresjo M., Carlsson E., Faresjo M., et al. 2014. "Psychological stress in children may alter the immune response". *Journal of Immunology*. 192 (5): 2071-2081.

32 McGonigal, Kelly. "How to make stress your friend." [September 2013] YouTube video, 14:28. https://www.youtube.com/watch?v=RcGyVTAoXEU

33 South Florida Public Broadcasting Station. "It's the Little Things: DailyRoutines." PBS.org https://www.pbs.org/wholechild/providers/little.html (accessed May 25, 2017)

34 Murray, Michael T., and Joseph E. Pizzorno. 2014. The encyclopedia of natural medicine.

PART III:
Basic Naturopathic Support for Illness

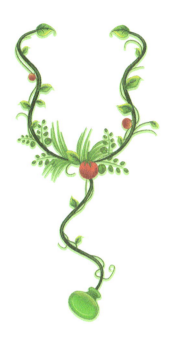

Children that grow and develop normally have certain habits in place: a healthy diet, regular exercise, sufficient sleep, healthy social interactions and stimulating mental activities. The focus of this chapter is the basic naturopathic support that can be used for any child during a time of illness, regardless of what the illness is. These particular therapies and remedies are fundamental and simple ways to take the best care of children's health. They enhance and stimulate immune function to increase natural killer cell, macrophage and T cell and B cell activity.

Chapter 4:
Basic Measures

Bed Rest

When the body is trying to mount an immune response, it diverts much of its resources to accomplishing that. By lying in bed and resting, we allow those resources to be used for fighting infection and re-establishing normal health. Bed rest should not include playing computer games or using tablets or phones. Watching a bit of television, reading and listening to soothing music are all acceptable activities. Remember, we tend to feel better before we are fully recovered. Allowing the body an extra 24-48 hours of rest, even after we think we are better, goes a long way to preventing relapse.

Fever

Many parents become concerned when their child has a fever. It is a sign that their child is not well. As scary as it can seem, it's important to note that while a fever is a sign of infection, that doesn't mean it needs to be stopped. So don't go to your medicine cabinet to find a fever reducer just yet.

Bacteria and viruses thrive at the regular body temperature of 98.6 degrees. When a fever is present, it indicates that the immune system is working correctly. Chemical messengers are being sent to stimulate the innate and adaptive parts of the immune system. These parts send out natural killer cells to kill bacteria and viruses and create antibodies. Without a fever, the immune system doesn't know it needs to take these steps.

There are many different types of fever. A slow, low-grade fever (99–101 degrees) is one where a child may still be happily playing and not seem bothered by it. A child with a higher temperature may not feel good (102–103 degrees) and may want to rest. When a fever rises quickly to a high temperature, 103+, it needs to be addressed because it can indicate a deeper state of infection.

Normally, children don't need to be treated for a high fever unless they're less than three months old. Febrile seizures happen because of a rapid change in temperature, not how high the temperature goes. Brain damage will not occur unless a fever is maintained at 107 degrees for a long period of time. Fevers can be supported by fluids, bed rest, keeping your child at a comfortable temperature and keeping cool rags on the head or on the body. It is no longer recommended by any health practitioner or organization to give a child any type of aspirin during a fever. It is also not advised to use a cold or ice water bath or alcohol rub.

Call your doctor when:

- ◆ your child's fever has continued at 104 degrees or more and has not responded to home treatment

- ◆ your child is less than three months old and has any fever

- ◆ your child is irritable and confused, has trouble breathing, has a stiff neck, has had a seizure or won't move an arm or leg.

When taking a child's temperature, use a temple thermometer and take it on both sides. Infants can have their temperature taken under the arm. (It is customary to add one to one and a half degrees if the temperature is taken under the arm.)

In general, it is important for parents and caregivers to realize that fever is a good thing. It's the body's way of self-regulating and restoring itself to health.

Food

When the body is trying to heal, the desire for food or exercise is not high. If a child does not want to eat, forcing a child to do so could hinder their healing capacity. Generally, it is a good idea to suspend daily supplements and allow the body's natural immunity to heal the body (It is customary to add one to one and a half degree to the thermometer reading if temperature is taken under the arm to know the actual temperature.)

If your child is hungry, there are certain foods that will provide energy without hindering the healing process. For example, oatmeal, rice, gluten-free toast, quinoa, amaranth cereal, raw veggies like celery, carrots, squashes, mushrooms and other assorted vegetables. Water (and herbal teas that are helpful for children) can be given as often as they like.

There are also certain foods to eliminate from your child's diet to promote healing. Dairy (including milk, cheese and yogurt), juices (all fruit and vegetable juices), fried foods, all processed foods (and anything that comes in a box, bag or package), sugar and sugary foods like cereal, cookies and desserts. Fruits should also be consumed at a minimum because of their high sugar content.

Chapter 5:
Edible Treatments

Broths

Rich in nutrients, easy on digestion and healing to the gut, broths have been used for centuries by healers. A broth is a water-based preparation to which is added a number of ingredients, mainly vegetables, herbs and sometimes meat. There is not much hard scientific evidence as to why broths have such a powerful impact on healing, but in our modern era a number of researchers have begun investigating how and why this nourishing liquid works.

One study found that good old fashioned chicken soup has a positive effect on the immune system.[1] It is believed that broth allows the body to shift focus from digesting solid foods to healing processes. One of the best advantages to using broths as part of the healing treatment is that they are inexpensive and can be made at home. Many holistic doctors actually recommend broths be a part of the regular diet.

Bone Broth

Bone broth was prepared by our ancestors using every part of an animal. Bones, marrow, skin, tendons and ligaments are all boiled over long periods. This releases a number of healing compounds such as collagen, proline, glycine and glutamine. Bone broth also contains minerals in forms that your body can easily absorb: calcium, magnesium, phosphorus, silicon, sulphur and others.

One important thing to keep in mind is that the broth is only as good as the ingredients used. Clean water, organic, grass-fed, free-range animals and organic vegetables are the best choices. Most store-bought bone broths are not the real thing, as manufacturers often use meat flavorings and may include ingredients such as monosodium glutamate (MSG), a neurotoxin. Also, most of the benefits of bone broth come from long-term consumption.

Bieler's Broth

Providing many of the same benefits as bone broth, this preparation is often made only with vegetables. Traditionally, the liquid is strained to be consumed and the vegetables are discarded to the compost pile.

Herbal Teas

Sometimes it can be challenging to get children to drink water. Because hydration is so important to health, a very nice way to keep them hydrated is to use herbal teas, most of which are naturally caffeine-free. Depending on the herbs you choose, you can also introduce a little bit of daily medicine to keep your child's immune system strong and vibrant. Children typically like colorful drinks and there are a number of herbs like rose hips, elderberry and hibiscus that will turn the drink pink, red or purple. The best sweeteners are raw honey or stevia. You can mix up a batch every few days and store in the fridge. They can be served cold or warm.

Ginger Tea

A flavorful tea, ginger is a widely used herb for medicinal benefits as well. It acts as an anti-inflammatory, stimulates circulation of blood, fights nausea, calms spasms, induces sweating and has mild antimicrobial effects. It is warming to the body and can noticeably affect digestion. For all these reason, it is an excellent herb to use as a tea to support the body during illness. A child that is less than a year old can easily have 3–4 tablespoons of tea. We listed ginger tea in this section because it can be used by any child at any age for any condition needing immune support. **Not all teas are appropriate for all conditions.**

The Home Tea Chest

While there are many herbs to choose from, and we talk about a number of different herbs in this book, there are several which can be consumed on a daily basis and which will provide nutritive as well as medicinal benefits. You can keep the following four herbs on hand and combine them to make a tea that can be served daily, warm or cold. We have included a recipe for "Everyday Herbal Tea" in the Apothecary section.

- Rose hips provide Vitamin C which can help restore and maintain healthy immune function. This will also lend a pinkish-red color to the tea.

- Lemon balm (*Melissa officinalis*) is a gentle green leaf herb that can support the nervous system, is calming, has immune supportive properties and tastes good. This makes a good base for any tea blend.

- Oatstraw (*Avena sativa*) is a nourishing herb that supports the general nervous system.

- Elderberry (*Sambucus nigra*) is a tasty herb that combines well with many herbs, especially the ones listed here. This herb supports the immune system, is anti-inflammatory, calming and can help keep mucous membranes clear.

Mushrooms

In general, many mushrooms contain a variety of substances that are considered to be medicinal and particularly important for supporting the immune system.[2] Chaga (*Inonotus obliquus*), cordyceps (*Ophiocordyceps sinensis*), reishi (*Ganoderma lucidum*) and shiitake (*Lentinula edodes*) mushrooms are most commonly thought of as having a direct effect on the immune function. While there are numerous preparations of mushrooms for little ones, the easiest way to consume medicinal mushrooms is as a glycerite.

Oxymels

Evidence dating from 460 BC[3] shows us this wonderful medicine has been used by doctors for a very long time to help stimulate healing in the human body. Traditionally, the base of the oxymel is honey and vinegar, to which many different herbs and medicines can be added. The key to using this successfully is to make it fresh and dose in small amounts frequently. Most commonly added for children are ginger, chamomile and lavender. It is believed that the oxymel can boost immune function, soothe inflammation and help the body detoxify from metabolic waste products produced when ill.

Probiotics

As a staple for children of all ages, probiotics stimulate immune function by affecting digestion, gut associated lymphatic vessels (the immune cells of the gut), mood and immunity. Probiotics are the microorganisms that affect our health positively by killing invasive bacteria that are harmful to health. The study of the benefits of probiotics within our digestive system continues to expand. Research is ongoing and continues to demonstrate new ways probiotics benefit our health.[4] They provide support to the lungs, skin, digestive organs, urinary tract and brain.[5] They are also safe to use from the time a child is born.[6]

During times of illness, higher amounts can be taken to stimulate immune function. Keep in mind that higher amounts of probiotics can affect bowel movements with either constipation or diarrhea occurring within hours after consuming them.

For babies that are breastfeeding, placing some powdered probiotics on the mother's nipples is sufficient. An infant that is not breastfeeding can have ⅛ teaspoon added to a room temperature beverage in a bottle. For children that are 1–5 years old, ¼–½ teaspoon of a children's probiotic is sufficient. Older children can easily handle ½ teaspoon or more per day. Watch for loose stools or constipation that can tell you it's too high of a dose.

1 Rennard, B. O., R. F. Ertl, G. L. Gossman, R. A. Robbins, and S. I. Rennard. 2000. "Chicken Soup Inhibits Neutrophil Chemotaxis In Vitro". CHEST -CHICAGO-. 118: 1150-1157.

2 Wasser, Solomon P. 2017. "Medicinal Mushrooms in Human Clinical Studies. Part I. Anticancer, Oncoimmunological, and Immunomodulatory Activities: A Review". *International Journal of Medicinal Mushrooms.* 19 (4): 279-317.

3 Zargaran A, MM Zarshenas, A Mehdizadeh, and A Mohagheghzadeh. 2012. "Oxymel in medieval Persia". *Pharmaceutical Historian.* 42 (1): 11-3.

Chapter 6:
Vitamins, Minerals & Supplements

Specific vitamins, minerals and supplements are safe and desirable during times of illness. They are agents for immune support when defenses are low.

Vitamin A

Vitamin A plays a critical role in human immunity. It is important to the normal function of cells such as natural killer (NK) cells, macrophages, neutrophils and T and B cells. Vitamin A can positively affect the outcome of childhood illnesses such as measles and pneumonia.[1,2] The dosing strategy is included in The Apothecary section.

It is important to note that vitamin A excess can happen when large amounts are taken over long periods of time. Symptoms of excess can include nausea, headache, fatigue, loss of appetite, dizziness, dry skin and swelling of the brain. It is rare for Vitamin A excess to develop when taking large amounts over a short period of time.

Vitamin C

The cells of the immune system need vitamin C to perform their task. Vitamin C deficiency can result in scurvy and a lower resistance to pathogens, while a high supply enhances immune function.[3] Vitamin C concentrations drop during times of stress and illness. It has been found that using this vitamin during illness can improve the body's ability to resist illness and recover.[4]

Vitamin C supplements are available but the best way to consume it is to use fresh whole foods (remember, cooking food can destroy the vitamin C in it). A small amount (varies depending on age) on an everyday basis helps keep the immune system strong. When used during illness, dosing small amounts frequently during the day is a good strategy for immune support.[5]

Vitamin D

Vitamin D is a nutrient that has numerous functions in the body. All our cells have receptors for it! It is especially important for young children because of its immune enhancing effects. Within the innate immune system, Vitamin D activates macrophages and monocytes (immune system killing agents), and induces antimicrobial peptides and reactive oxygen species which kill microorganisms. It affects the adaptive immune system by activating T cells (stimulating the production of cells that will kill microorganisms) and B cells (which support antibody creation).[6]

Zinc

Zinc is a commonly used mineral during times of illness. When treating colds, it binds to the receptors that viruses would attach to inhibiting their ability to continue to reproduce in the body.[7] When combating diarrhea, some of the ways it helps is by regulating fluid transport and maintaining the integrity of the gastrointestinal lining.[8] In cases of pneumonia, it competes with the minerals that bacteria need to survive, essentially starving them to death.[9] When looking at overall immune function, studies show that zinc increases phagocytosis (process by which immune cells eat foreign invaders), positively enhances the activity of T cell (immune helper cells) and B cells (antibodies), as well as increasing different types of immune system cells. In addition, it acts as an antioxidant and plays a role in hundreds of metabolic pathways in the body.[10]

Iodine

When people think of iodine they usually associate it with the thyroid gland. Research, however, has established that iodine can also be used as an antimicrobial to quickly kill bacteria, viruses, fungi and various other organisms.[11] While special preparations of iodine can be taken internally, one of the safest, simplest and most effective ways to use it is when addressing an acute illness to mix it with a carrier oil, such as coconut oil, and massage it into lymph nodes.

N-acetyl Cysteine (NAC)

NAC is a modified version of the amino acid cysteine. When taken internally, NAC can increase levels of glutathione (GSH), an antioxidant which helps protect cell from free radicals. Even though it has been used in conventional medicine for over thirty years for a variety of purposes including as a mucous thinner, many doctors know little about it. Among its many benefits and uses, NAC has been proven highly effective against influenza and influenza-like illnesses.[12] It can reduce the length and severity of illness as well as protect against the more serious complications that can develop in the very young and elderly.[13] Because it can increase levels of glutathione, it is likely that scientists will continue to discover the benefits of NAC over time. For the purposes of this book, anytime mucous production is present as part of an illness, including NAC with other treatments can be very beneficial.

1 Huiming Y, W Chaomin, and M Meng. 2005. "Vitamin A for treating measles in children". The Cochrane Database of Systematic Reviews. 2005 (4).

2 "American Academy of Pediatrics Committee on Infectious Diseases: Vitamin A treatment of measles". 1993. Pediatrics. 91 (5): 1014-5.

3 Ströhle A, and A Hahn. 2009. "Vitamin C und Immunfunktion". Medizinische Monatsschrift Fur Pharmazeuten. 32 (2): 49-54.

4 Wintergerst, E. S., S. Maggini, and D. H. Hornig. 2006. "Immune-Enhancing Role of Vitamin C and Zinc and Effect on Clinical Conditions". ANNALS OF NUTRITION AND METABOLISM. 50 (2): 85-94.

5 Jariwalla RJ, and S Harakeh. 1996. "Antiviral and immunomodulatory activities of ascorbic acid". Sub-Cellular Biochemistry. 25: 213-31.

6 Bikle, Daniel D. 2014. "Vitamin D Metabolism, Mechanism of Action, and Clinical Applications". Chemistry & Biology. 21(3), 319-329.

7 Novick, S.G., J.C. Godfrey, N.J. Godfrey, and H.R. Wilder. 1996. "How does zinc modify the common cold? Clinical observations and implications regarding mechanisms of action". Medical Hypotheses. 46 (3): 295-302.

8 Canani R.B., Buccigrossi V., and Passariello A. 2011. "Mechanisms of action of zinc in acute diarrhea". Current Opinion in Gastroenterology. 27 (1): 8-12.

9 McDevitt CA, AD Ogunniyi, E Valkov, MC Lawrence, B Kobe, AG McEwan, and JC Paton. 2011. "A molecular mechanism for bacterial susceptibility to zinc". PLoS Pathogens. 7 (11).

10 Prasad, A.S. 2008. "Zinc in Human Health: Effect of Zinc on Immune Cells". MOLECULAR MEDICINE -CAMBRIDGE MA THEN NEW YORK-. 14 (5/6): 353-357.

11 Iodine Research Resource Network of The Iodine Movement. "Iodine and the Body Immune System." iodineresearch.com. http://iodineresearch.com (accessed Aug 25, 2017).

12 Geiler, Janina, Martin Michaelis, Patrizia Naczk, Anke Leutz, Klaus Langer, Hans-Wilhelm Doerr, and Jindrich Cinatl. 2010. "N-acetyl-l-cysteine (NAC) inhibits virus replication and expression of pro-inflammatory molecules in A549 cells infected with highly pathogenic H5N1 influenza A virus". Biochemical Pharmacology. 79 (3): 413-420.

13 De Flora, S., C. Grassi, and L. Carati. 1997. "Attenuation of influenza-like symptomatology and improvement of cell-mediated immunity with long-term N-acetylcysteine treatment". EUROPEAN RESPIRATORY JOURNAL. 10 (7): 1535-1541.

Chapter 7:
Physical & Environmental Remedies

Hydrotherapy

As mentioned previously, there are numerous forms of hydrotherapy treatments that you can easily and safely do at home or can safely be administered by a naturopathic doctor.

Constitutional Hydrotherapy

Constitutional hydrotherapy is another water-based therapy that enhances overall well-being. It causes superficial blood vessels in the skin to dilate and then contract. The contraction of superficial blood vessels floods blood into internal organs allowing them access to new oxygenated blood and increased white blood cells.

First, you must wrap your child in a wool blanket and have them lie down. Then use alternating hot and cold towels, applied over longer periods of time while applying a sine wave machine to gently provide electrical stimulation. The increased circulation brings more nutrients, oxygen and white blood cells to internal organs. It also allows the immune system to actively work while a child rests. Many children fall asleep or feel deeply relaxed after this treatment is completed.

Contrast Hydrotherapy

This therapy works through the placement of hot and cold towels over the chest and abdomen. When hot towels are placed on the body, superficial blood vessels dilate, bringing more blood to the surface of the body. When cold towels are applied to the chest and abdomen, the superficial blood vessels constrict, causing blood to rapidly flow into internal organs. This action pumps more blood into the organs and directly acts on the thymus gland to increase output of white blood cells. The towels should be placed in alternating succession, hot towels first and cold towels last, to promote this immune response. The secondary effect seen is a deep relaxation which helps children's body naturally go into a repair state.

Medicinal Baths

These baths can be used to relax or cool down a child as well as support a healing response in the body. Essential oils of lavender or chamomile can be placed in a bath to help calm down a child (just a few drops is plenty). A cool (but not cold) bath can make a child with a fever more comfortable without stopping the immune benefits of said fever. A bath with herbs (oats, lavender, comfrey or calendula) can be soothing to the skin and relaxing to the nervous system.

Caution: It's important not to place a child with a fever in a cold bath because the change in temperature can be a shock to the body, potentially starting a seizure. A child with a high fever should be cooled with cool wet washcloths or towels.

Washcloth Hydrotherapy

Since babies have smaller torsos, a cool washcloth can be placed over the chest and abdomen to keep them comfortable if they have a fever. Also, alternating warm and cool washcloths can help increase circulation thereby increasing immune function. This works in the same way as contrast hydrotherapy. Since very young babies do not control their temperatures very well and have very sensitive skin in the first few weeks of life, it is not recommended to use very hot or very cold washcloths on their bodies.

Steam inhalations

This therapy involves breathing in steam of a medicated water that has essential oils in it or just water alone. Essential oils are suggested because of the immune-stimulating effects they have. Steam inhalations are generally used by people that have upper respiratory conditions like stuffy noses or congested sinuses. One to two drops of essential oils are sufficient for a child.

Massage and Brushing

Dry Skin Brushing

The use of a dry skin brush is meant to support lymphatic circulation and removal of old, dead cells from the body. Since lymphatic vessels are superficial, light brushing strokes moving towards the heart are the easiest way to move lymphatic fluid. The lymphatic system does not have its own pump so helping it move either through exercise or dry skin brushing is something that can safely be done by children (and adults) of all ages.

Lymphatic massage

The touch of a loved one goes a long way toward helping a child feel cared for.The gentle, soft touch of a lymphatic massage can help an ill child remove metabolic waste products and dead cells from the lymphatic system. The bond shared through touch extends beyond the physical plane and into the heart where nerve signals allow your child to relax and allow healing to naturally occur. Remember, lymphatic vessels are fairly superficial so a light touch is all that is needed to support the body through illness.

Socks

Garlic socks

This treatment is used to stimulate the immune system without the need for children to consume garlic. Garlic has antimicrobial effects, strengthens the immune system and fights inflammation. For this treatment, smashed garlic is applied through a cheesecloth onto a child's foot and socks are placed over them (only one clove of garlic is needed). They can be left on during a nap or overnight. In the morning, your child's breath may smell like garlic because of absorption of garlic constituents through the feet.

Magic Socks

Considered to be a type of hydrotherapy, magic socks can stimulate the immune system, drain congestion from the head and chest, relax away aches, increase circulation and aid in detoxification. The exact process is outlined in the Apothecary section.

PART IV:
The Conditions

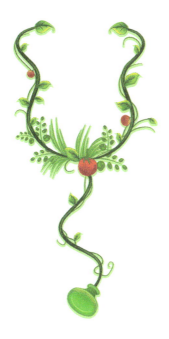

This section covers the descriptions of common childhood illnesses for which vaccinations are available, and as of 2017, are part of the CDC vaccination schedule (except for the flu). Statistics were taken from the CDC's publicly available records. Included are transmission routes, infection rates and disease prevalence. Possible complications from each illness is discussed. Each condition includes the vitalistic naturopathic approach as well as the herbs, supplements, essential oils, homeopathic remedies and other therapies that are best indicated.

Chapter 8:
Chickenpox (Varicella)

Varicella zoster, commonly known as chickenpox, belongs to the herpesvirus family. It is a contagious virus which occurs most commonly in winter and spring. Before routine vaccination started in the mid-1990s, it affected children of all ages, primarily younger children. There were up to 3.5 million cases per year. Today we see about 700,000 cases nationwide. It can have severe complications for children younger than one year of age,[1] and resulted in about 150 deaths per year. Today, we see about thirty deaths per year in immunocompromised children, such as children with HIV.

The primary route of infection is airborne via respiratory droplets, through the conjunctiva or direct contact with infected skin from chickenpox lesions (fluid-filled blisters).

A chickenpox infection is usually mild but risks and complications from chickenpox can include a bacterial infection at the site of a blister from scratching or pneumonia. If it enters the central nervous system, it can lead to meningitis or encephalitis. If it reaches the brain, it can affect the cerebellum (coordinates movement and speech) and recovery from this type of infection, generally, comes easily. Rarely, it can affect internal organs like the liver and spleen.[2]

If exposed, susceptible adults, pregnant women, immunocompromised children and neonates can receive injection of varicella-zoster immune globulin (VZIG) within seventy-two hours to prevent infection or decrease severity. Giving VZIG to pregnant moms will not protect a fetus from a possible infection.

The incubation period for chickenpox is 14–16 days after exposure. There may be a mild fever (99-102 degrees) and general sense of not feeling well before the rash, but the rash is often the first sign of disease. It usually starts on the head, chest and back, and then spreads to the rest of the body. The rash typically starts as raised pink or red bumps (papules), which break out over several days and eventually develop into blisters. These blisters will break and leak a bit of fluid, then scab over and fall off.

New papules continue to appear for several days and throughout the week your child may have all three kinds of eruptions—papules, blisters and scabs—at the same time. Frequently there will be fatigue, itchiness, loss of appetite and irritability during the week of the rash. After about 5–6 days, the scabs fall off leaving freshly healed skin. Your child is contagious from forty-eight hours before the rash appears until all the blisters have all scabbed over and fallen off.

There is no conventional medical treatment for chickenpox. Doctors will prescribe topical creams to relieve itching. If exposed, they may prescribe antiviral medications but they are only given to otherwise healthy children older than twelve years of age.[3]

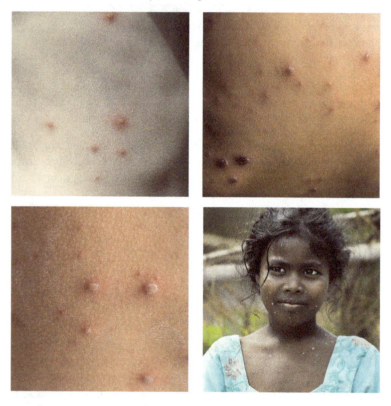

Vitalistic Naturopathic Approach

Basic naturopathic support includes bed rest, broths, oxymel, vitamin A, C and D, zinc, ginger tea, probiotics, garlic or magic socks, dry skin brushing, medicinal baths, hydrotherapy, lymphatic massage, steam inhalation, mushrooms and NAC. If you haven't already reviewed Part 3, that is the section where we discuss these therapies at length.

Keep in mind that the skin may be very sensitive to touch and if so, adjust the therapies with your child's comfort in mind. Abstain from scratching lesions. Use homeopathic and/or topical medication to soothe itching and irritation. The following suggestions are specific for working with chickenpox.

Herbs

- Nettles (*Urtica dioica*) as a tea or glycerite soothes itchiness.

- Lemon balm (*Melissa officinalis*) as a tea or glycerite acts as a mild pain reliever, has antiviral effects, eases anxiety by calming the nervous system.

- Burdock (*Arctium lappa*) as a tea or a base for a soup helps skin recover and heal more quickly.

- Antiviral herbs (viral meningitis) such as elderberry (*Sambucus nigra*), astragalus (*Astragalus membranaceus*), echinacea (*Echinacea angustifolia* and/or *Echinacea purpurea*), osha (*Ligusticum porteri*) can be consumed as glycerites.

Supplements

- Lysine powder, in apple or pear sauce, acts as antiviral support.

- Vitamin A flush. This is a treatment that can be highly effective but should be done under the supervision of a naturopathic physician or other qualified health care practitioner.

Essential Oils

Essential oils can help address the underlying viral infection that causes chickenpox as well as soothe the itching.

- *Ravensara aromatica* has strong antiviral activity.[4]

- German chamomile (*Matricaria chamomilla*) soothes skin irritation and itching.

- Tea tree (*Melaleuca alternifolia*) also has antiviral effects and is helpful to soothe any skin irritation.

- Lavender (*Lavandula angustifolia*) soothes the skin, reduces itching, and has mild antiviral effects. Lavender also has a calming effect which can be very helpful for children suffering with itching and other symptoms.

You can use this combination of three essential oils in the bath:

+ Two drops each of ravensara, German chamomile (or lavender), and tea tree essential oils to one tablespoon of milk (cow, goat, almond, coconut, hemp, etc.) The oil and protein in the milk helps to disperse the essential oil in the bathwater. Avoid adding essential oils directly to the bathwater. They do not disperse and can cause skin irritation. Add to a warm bath and soak as long as desired.

+ Create an oil to rub into the skin. If you are an adult applying the oil to a child's skin, use latex-free gloves to avoid contaminating yourself and others.

+ Add two drops of ravensara, German chamomile, and tea tree essential oils to a tablespoon of pure, organic vegetable oil. Rub into the skin 3–4 times a day. Rub the oil first into the soles of the feet; then into the affected areas.

+ For children under six years old, dilute the essential oils in two tablespoons of pure, organic vegetable oil.

Homeopathy

A child with chickenpox may have a mild fever (99–102 degrees) and general sense of not feeling well followed by a rash, but the rash is often the first sign of disease. The rash starts as pink or raised bumps on the head, chest and back, and then spreads to the rest of the body. It eventually develops into blisters. The remedies listed here describe additional unique symptoms your child may have.

The easiest way to choose the remedy you think may work is to compare the list of symptoms you have made for your child to those listed under each remedy. Pick the one that seems to be the best match. For more explanation on how to create a list of symptoms, refer to the homeopathy section in Part 2 of this book.

The following remedies are the most common for this condition but keep in mind that the best remedy for your child may not be listed here. If you're having difficulty choosing a remedy, consider working with a homeopathic or naturopathic doctor to choose the best remedy.

◆ **Variolinum/Varicella (Vario/Varic) 30C**

Used in the homeopathic prophylactic protocol to help reduce the risk and severity of symptoms.

◆ **Antimonium crudum (Ant-c) 30C**

The child is irritable and may object or cry when touched or looked at. The pox are sore with shooting pains when touched. They look scaly, full of pus, burn, itch and all these symptoms are worse at night.

◆ **Apis mellifica (Apis) 30C**

The skin around the pox is pink, puffy and very itchy, with stinging pains. The eyelids may also be swollen. The child feels worse from warmth, is irritable and usually is not thirsty.

◆ **Bryonia (Bry) 30C**

When fever persists for several days during chickenpox, and a dry, painful nagging cough develops, this remedy may be useful. The child's mouth is dry and they are thirsty for cold drinks. The child may be very irritable and is almost always worse from motion. They prefer to lie still and do not want to be bothered in any way. The symptoms are all worse with warmth and motion (this is opposite of Rhus-t where the symptoms are better with warmth and motion).

◆ **Mercurius solubilis (Merc) 30C**

In Merc, the pox are large and become infected. The child is very sensitive to temperature changes and feels worse at night. There is much perspiration and drooling during sleep. The child's lymph nodes are typically swollen and their breath is foul.

◆ **Rhus tox (Rhus-t) 30C**

This is a common remedy for chickenpox and when the symptoms match it works incredibly fast to bring relief. There is often intense itching with great restlessness and these symptoms are worse at night and when the child has to be still. The child has difficulty going to and staying asleep due to the itching. They may thrash about the bed trying to get comfortable. The pox are large and incredibly itchy and feel worse from scratching. They are better with heat like a hot pack. The pox may have clear or pus-filled fluid. The child's muscles can ache and feel very stiff and these symptoms may also be better from warmth and motion. This is a very good remedy for the itchy phases.

 ♦ **Sulphur (Sulph) 30C**

If itching is so severe that the child finds it impossible to keep from scratching—or if the pox have a nagging, burning pain—and heat makes everything worse, Sulph may be the best remedy. The symptoms (and the child) become worse from warmth and after bathing. They can have both heat and chills during the fever. The child may feel drowsy in the afternoon and restless and hot at night. The itching is much worse in bed at night.

 ♦ **Urtica urens (Urt-u) 30C**

The pox itch violently with a crawling sensation, burning and stinging pains. There may be red blotches on the skin around the pox and aching in the joints.

 ♦ Additional remedies to consider for chickenpox include: Ant-t, Carb-v, Puls and Sepia.

Other Therapies

The following therapies can be used to support healing from this condition.

 ♦ Burdock (*Arctium lappa*) poultice to soothe the skin.

 ♦ Calendula (*Calendula officinalis*) wash to help heal skin and reduce scarring

 ♦ Soaking bath with baking soda, cornstarch, or milky oats to soothe the skin.

 ♦ Aloe vera gel, chickweed (*Stellaria media*) poultice, lavender (*Lavandula spp.*) poultice or oil topically soothe the skin.

 ♦ Dietary considerations: Temporarily reduce arginine-containing foods during outbreak such as dairy, spirulina, chocolate, peas, lentils, nuts and seeds, pork, turkey and chicken. Foods high in arginine can throw off the lysine-arginine balance in the body. Higher amounts of arginine can stimulate viral reproduction.[5, 6]

1 Lopez MHS, Adriana, Scott Schmid, PhD, Stephanie Bialek, MD, MPH. "Manual for the Surveillance of Vaccine-Preventable Diseases Chapter 17: Varicella." cdc.gov. https://www.cdc.gov/vaccines/pubs/surv-manual/chpt17-varicella.html (accessed February 1, 2017).

2 Centers for Disease Control and Prevention. "Epidemiology and Prevention of Vaccine-Preventable Diseases, 13th Edition Varicella" cdc.gov. https://www.cdc.gov/vaccines/pubs/pinkbook/downloads/varicella.pdf (accessed February 1, 2017).

3 Centers for Disease Control and Prevention. "Chickenpox (Varicella) Prevention & Treatment." cdc.gov. https://www.cdc.gov/chickenpox/about/prevention-treatment.html (accessed February 1, 2017).

4 Price, Shirley, and Len Price. 2015. *Aromatherapy for health professionals.* Edinburgh [etc.]: Churchill Livingstone. 90-91

5 Griffith, Richard S., Arthur L. Norins, and Christopher Kagan. 2004. "A Multicentered Study of Lysine Therapy in Herpes simplex Infection". *Dermatology.* 156 (5): 257-267.

6 Griffith, Richard S., Donald C. DeLong, and Janet D. Nelson. 2004. "Relation of Arginine-Lysine Antagonism to Herpes simplex Growth in Tissue Culture". *Chemotherapy.* 27 (3): 209-213.

Chapter 9:
Diphtheria

Diphtheria used to be widespread in the U.S. during the autumn and winter months, before the 1940s when universal immunizations were implemented. From 2004–2015, the U.S. reported two cases of diphtheria. As of 2016, the World Health Organization (WHO) reported just over 7,300 cases worldwide in places like Eastern Europe, Southeast Asia, Africa, the Caribbean and Latin America. The children affected were less than five years old.[1]

Diphtheria is a contagious bacterial illness, caused by the *Corynebacterium diphtheriae* bacterium. It is spread by coughing, sneezing and direct exposure through physical contact with infected objects, like toys. Parents and physicians were concerned about this illness because of the pseudomembrane that would grow as the bacteria released a toxin that killed off healthy lung tissue, obstructing normal breathing. This membrane could also cover the nose and throat and cause extensive swelling in the glands of the neck, making it difficult to breathe and swallow. If the toxin entered into the bloodstream, it could damage the kidneys, heart and nerves.

The signs and symptoms of diphtheria usually come on slowly over 2–5 days and often start with a sore throat, hoarseness, nasal discharge, fever and/or chills and a general overall sense of not feeling well. In severe and late stage cases, a thick, gray membrane may develop, covering the throat and tonsils. This can be accompanied by enlarged lymph nodes in the neck and difficult or rapid breathing. The duration of this condition is typically 7–10 days although in an immunocompromised individual it can last much longer.

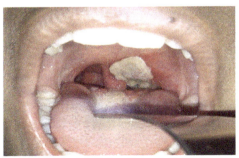

Photo credit: http://www.nigeriagalleria.com/Community-Health/Diphtheria.html

The conventional medical treatment for diphtheria is antibiotics. To date, it is responsive to this treatment.

Vitalistic Naturopathic Approach

A soft diet (to promote easier swallowing) and strict bed rest is suggested if your child is diagnosed with diphtheria. Basic naturopathic support includes bed rest, broths, oxymel, vitamin A, C and D, zinc, ginger tea, probiotics, garlic or magic socks, medicinal baths, hydrotherapy, dry skin brushing, lymphatic massage, steam inhalation, mushrooms and NAC. If you haven't already reviewed Part 3, that is the section where we discuss these therapies at length. The following suggestions are specific for working with diphtheria:

Herbs

♦ Garlic (*Allium sativum*) taken internally or used as a gargle. Internal use is most effective with freshly peeled/chopped garlic. For children, some of the most palatable ways to get in garlic is as a Garlic Oxymel, as a Ginger-Garlic tea, in Immune Soup or as a spread on toast. It can also be used as a Garlic Gargle. Look in the recipe section for all of the above. Another use for children that don't like the taste of garlic is to do a Garlic Socks treatment.

♦ Berberine containing antibacterial herbs: goldenseal (*Hydrastis canadensis*), barberry (*Berberis vulgaris*), Oregon grape root (*Mahonia aquifolium*), coptis (*Coptis chinensis*). Because of their taste, they are best consumed as glycerites. Although these are not discussed in botanical medical literature as being specific to diphtheria, they are general antibacterial herbs. Choose one of these herbs.

♦ Lavender (*Lavandula angustifolia*) used as a tea or topically as a lavender infused oil. This herb does not have any direct action on *C. diphtheriae*; however, it does reduce pain, inflammation and spasm and can help make a child more comfortable.

♦ Lomatium (*Lomatium dissectum*) used as a tea or glycerite, is a strong antimicrobial (bacteria and viruses) herb and has an affinity for the lungs. It stimulates the production of white blood cells and is immunomodulating. It enhances the production and release of mucus and eases spasms connected to cough. It is also a nutritive herb that supports the body during long-standing illness.

- Yerba Santa (*Eriodictyon californicum/ Eriodictyon angustifolium*) as a tea is used for upper respiratory infections when there is a lot of mucus production. It eases cough, opens up the airways, has antimicrobial (bacteria and viruses) effects, acts as a decongestant, breaks up mucus, and eases coughing spasms.

- Elecampane (*Inula helenium*) as a glycerite assists with expectoration, reduces inflammation, is warming to the lungs and is a lung tonic. It has antibacterial, antiviral and antifungal effects.

Supplements

- Vitamin A flush: This is a treatment that can be highly effective but should be done under the supervision of a naturopathic physician or other qualified health care practitioner.

- Mushroom formula containing a blend of chaga (*Inonotus obliquus*), cordyceps (*Ophiocordyceps sinensis*), reishi (*Ganoderma lucidum*) and shiitake (*Lentinula edodes*). Used as a glycerite or in apple or pear sauce, mushrooms strengthen and support immune function.

- Manuka honey added to rooibos tea to soothe the throat and promote healing in the tissue.

Essential Oils

- *Eucalyptus radiata* is used during the early stages of diphtheria as a steam inhalation. It is a wonderful ally to reduce congestion and address the infection.

- Tea tree (*Melaleuca alternifolia*) is especially useful as a gargle. It has antibacterial properties and is safe even for very young children.

- Utilized via a topical application (rubbed into soles of feet, on chest and on throat), the following essential oils have been researched and found to have specific antibacterial activity for diphtheria.[2] Choose 1–2 of the following oils and repeat application every 2–3 hours.

    - Coriander (*Coriandrum sativum*)

    - Lavender (*Lavandula angustifolia*)

- Tea tree (*Melaleuca alternifolia*)

- Rosemary (*Rosmarinus officinalis*)

Homeopathy

A child with diphtheria will likely have some or all of the general symptoms including a sore throat, hoarseness, nasal discharge, fever and/ or chills, swollen lymph nodes and a general overall sense of not feeling well. In addition to these, you will notice that there are more specific qualities that may be unique to what your child is experiencing. The remedies listed here describe unique symptoms your child may have.

The easiest way to choose the remedy you think may work is to compare the list of symptoms you have made for your child to those listed under each remedy. Pick the one that seems to be the best match. For more explanation on how to create a list of symptoms, refer to the homeopathy section in Part 2 of this book.

The following remedies are the most common for this condition but keep in mind that the best remedy for your child may not be listed here. If you're having difficulty choosing a remedy, consider working with a homeopathic or naturopathic doctor to choose the best remedy.

- **Diphtherinum (Diph) 30C:**

    Used in the homeopathic prophylactic protocol to help reduce the risk and severity of symptoms.

- **Lachesis (Lach) 30C**

    Extreme sensitivity of the throat is present: sensitive to swallowing, sensitive to touch, sensitive to tight things around the neck. Symptoms often appear first on the left side of the throat and then spread to the right. There is often extremely painful and difficult swallowing, violent prostration and bad odor coming from the throat. In general, the child or the child's symptoms are worse on awakening from sleep, even naps. The throat can be a purplish color with much swelling inside and out. A striking symptom is that the throat feels worse from empty swallowing (swallowing spit).

- **Baptisia (Bapt) 30C**

    Bapt may be needed if there is septic (bacterial) poisoning, foul odor, feverish (hot) breath, dark red tissues in the throat, painful swelling of glands, aching of back. The body and limbs may hurt as if pounded. The face is dark red, flushed like they have ingested a poison and the tongue is dry and redder than normal. The striking symptoms are the dryness of the mouth accompanied by great thirst and the child is much worse with ANY movement and prefers to be completely still.

◆ Lycopodium (Lyc) 30C

Symptoms often start on the right side of the throat and can spread to the left (opposite of Lach in which symptoms start on the left and move to the right). Pain is worse on the right side of throat. There may be stoppage (congestion) of the nose, with inability to breathe through it. You may notice the child flaring the edges of their nostrils. The child can be worse after sleeping and after swallowing drinks, especially cold ones. Symptoms seem to be worse from 4–8 PM and then there is a slight improvement. In general, any child needing Lyc may have tummy troubles which include loud rumblings and an increase in passing gas.

◆ Lac caninum (Lac-c) 30C

There is often swelling of the throat both internally and externally. The child is extremely restless. The child may be urinating much less than normal. A striking symptom is that the pains may alternate sides in either of the following patterns: moving right-left-right or left-right-left.

◆ Kali bichromicum (Kali-b) 30C

Deep ulcerations of the tissue may be present. All of their expectorations or other discharges can be very thick, sticky or stringy, yellowish and may be streaked with blood. The membrane in the throat, if present, is more yellow than gray. There may be a croup-like cough with pains in the chest that extend to the neck and shoulders. Hard swelling of the glands may be present. The tongue is often yellow-coated or very dry and red. This remedy is often indicated in late or croupid stages (spasmodic laryngitis with a cough and difficulty breathing). One of the most striking symptoms for this remedy is the thick, sticky, stringy and yellow colored discharges.

- **Kali muriaticum (Kali-m) 30C**

  There is pain on swallowing and a milky white deposit in the throat. This remedy can be helpful for the croupid form of disease. In the literature, these are the main symptoms prescribed on but numerous cases of the disease have been treated with the remedy and symptoms like prostration, thick discharge over the tonsils and entire soft palate, foul breath, etc., have entirely disappeared.

- **Kali permanganicum (Kali-perm) 30C**

  Ulceration of the tissues with gangrenous pus producing discharge and extremely foul odor is seen. Swelling of the throat occurs both internally and externally. If there is a membrane present it smells horribly offensive. There can be a thin discharge from the nose and difficult swallowing.

- **Apis mellifica (Apis) 30C**

  A common appearance for children who need Apis is a red swelling with stinging pains and a sore blistered tongue. The throat may have a glossy-red appearance. If there is a membrane that forms, it can be on either tonsil and is grayish, dirty-looking and tough. The child can have a very difficult time swallowing. They may complain that they are completely exhausted and feel weak but seem to be restless and moving about. The skin can be dry and hot and the amount of urine is decreased. The striking symptoms with this remedy are the red swelling and stinging pains.

- **Phytolacca (Phyt) 30C**

  The pains in the throat shoot outward into the ears or downward into the neck. The glands of the neck and behind the ears become hard and inflamed. There can be inflammation of the throat with an accumulation of thick, sticky mucus. The tonsils can be quite swollen, almost to the point where it appears they touch one another. The child or the child's symptoms may be worse at night, on cold days, in a cold room and from the heat of the bed. Striking symptoms of this remedy are: great swellings of the throat or tonsils, swelling of the glands of the neck, aching in the bones, foul odor from the mouth with heavily coated tongue, great aching in the back, nosebleeds and soreness of the muscles.

Other Therapies

The following therapies can be used to support healing from this condition.

- Contrast hydrotherapy to the neck. This therapy stimulates local immune function and circulation.

- Iodine rub to the neck to support local immune function.

- Saltwater and colloidal silver gargle: two years or older (must be able to gargle) to help reduce inflammation and infection.

- Eucalyptus steam inhalation[3] to help reduce inflammation and infection.

1 Centers for Disease Control and Prevention. "Diphtheria Clinicians." cdc.gov. https://www.cdc.gov/diphtheria/clinicians.html (accessed February 1, 2017).

2 Price, Shirley, and Len Price. 2015. Aromatherapy for health professionals. Edinburgh [etc.]: Churchill Livingstone. 76-78

3 The Epitome of medicine A monthly retrospect of progress in all divisions of medico-chirurgical practice. ... Vol. I-X, [1884-1893]. 1884. New York: G.P. Putnam's Sons.

Chapter 10:
Flu (Influenza)

Influenza, more commonly known as the flu, is a condition that comes to the forefront of the public's mind every year in late fall and winter as news about it starts circulating. Influenza is a contagious mild to severe respiratory illness caused by a number of different influenza viruses. Symptoms of the flu include fever, cough, runny nose, sore throat, muscle aches and pains, weakness, fatigue and headache.[1]

In some cases, the flu can cause complications like ear and sinus infections, bronchitis and pneumonia. Young children are considered higher risk because of their underdeveloped immune system. If a child less than five years old experiences trouble breathing, bluish skin color, is highly irritable, not interacting with others, not waking up or seem to improve then get much worse, they need further medical assistance. An infant that is not eating, has fewer wet diapers, no tears when crying and is having trouble breathing requires medical attention. In rare instances, death can be a result of the flu.[2]

From 2015–2016, there were sporadic cases of the flu throughout the United States with the majority of cases in New York state, New Jersey, Pennsylvania, New England and Kentucky. There were seven strains of the flu circulating during that time. Eighteen strains of the flu were found to be resistant to antiviral medications. There were eighty-five pediatric deaths in that timeframe.[3]

The number of flu cases are reported weekly by state. A quick check on the CDC website can give you more information about what's happening in your local area.

Generally, a person that gets the flu will recover within a few days or a couple weeks. Conventional medicine currently does not have any treatments available.

Vitalistic Naturopathic Approach

Basic naturopathic support includes bed rest, broths, oxymel, vitamin A, C and D, zinc, ginger tea, probiotics, garlic or magic socks, medicinal baths, hydrotherapy, dry skin brushing, lymphatic massage, steam inhalation, mushrooms and NAC. If you haven't already reviewed Part

3, that is the section where we discuss these therapies at length. The following suggestions are specific for working with the flu.

Herbs

- Ginger (*Zingiber officinale*) as a tea can address nausea, vomiting and ease pain.

- Elderberry (*Sambucus nigra*) is best taken as a syrup or glycerite. It is a general immune tonic increasing white blood cell activity and has antimicrobial effects.

- Astragalus (*Astragalus membranaceus*) is best taken as a syrup or glycerite. It is an adaptogenic herb which restores normal function, has anti-inflammatory and antiviral effects and is an immunomodulator.

- Echinacea (*Echinacea angustifolia* and/or *Echinacea purpurea*) as a tincture or glycerite is supportive to the immune system and has antimicrobial effects.

- Lomatium (*Lomatium dissectum*) used as a tea or glycerite is a strong antimicrobial (bacteria and viruses) and has an affinity for the lungs. It stimulates the production of white blood cells, is immunomodulating, enhances the production and release of mucus, and eases spasms connected to cough. It is also a nutritive that supports the body during long-standing illness.

Supplements

- Vitamin A flush: This is a treatment that can be highly effective but should be done under the supervision of a naturopathic physician or other qualified health care practitioner.

Essential Oils

Inhaling essential oils rapidly delivers healing support to the respiratory system, and through absorption in the lungs, to the entire body. For ALL essential oils: avoid using a cold diffuser that runs continuously. Long-term (e.g. more than 45–60 minutes), ongoing exposure to any essential oil stresses the liver's detoxification pathways, particularly for young children. Ongoing exposures also increases the risk of sensitizing your child to that essential oil in particular and to essential oils in general. In this condition, essential oils quickly address the virus itself and provide relief for the uncomfortable symptoms.

An essential oil found to be effective against the H2N2 (pandemic) influenza:

- Patchouli (*Pogostemon cablin*)[4]

- *Ravensara aromatica* has strong antiviral activity[5]

- *Eucalyptus radiata* helps to open the bronchi, expectorate mucus, and reduce inflammation

- Rosemary (*Rosmarinus officinalis*) ct verbenone has mucolytic action

- Bay laurel (*Laurus nobilis*) helps to expectorate mucus

Chest and foot rub: Choose from the essential oils listed above. Rotate the combination of essential oils you are using every 2–3 days, to avoid the skin becoming sensitized to the essential oils.

Inhalation: Choose one or a combination of the above essential oils. Test the oils first on a tissue and inhale to make sure you like the smell of the combination (if your nose is clear enough to smell!) You will have benefit from the essential oils, even if you have no sense of smell. If you can smell, you will be more likely to use the inhaler if you enjoy the scent.

Homeopathy

A child with the flu may have symptoms such as fever and chills, cough, muscle aches (especially in back, arms and legs) and a headache. There can be nausea and vomiting and a sore throat or chest pains accompanied by a cough and difficulty breathing. The remedies listed here describe additional unique symptoms your child may have.

The easiest way to choose the remedy you think may work is to compare the list of symptoms you have made for your child to those listed under each remedy. Pick the one that seems to be the best match. For more explanation on how to create a list of symptoms, refer to the homeopathy section in Part 2 of this book.

The following remedies are the most common for this condition but keep in mind that the best remedy for your child may not be listed here. If you're having difficulty choosing a remedy, consider working with a homeopathic or naturopathic doctor to choose the best remedy.

Prophylactic remedies to help reduce risk (can use any or all):

- **Influenzinum 30C (current year):**

    Used in the homeopathic prophylactic protocol to help reduce the risk and severity of symptoms.

- **Oscillococcinum:**

    As a preventative at the beginning of flu season,[6,7]

    If symptoms of the flu are present:

- **Arsenicum Album (Ars) 30C**

    You will notice symptoms of chill, weakness, restlessness and anxiety. The child will be thirsty for frequent sips of cold water. Discharges from a blocked and stuffy nose will be thin and watery. The child and symptoms will be worse from cold air, cold applications and from 1:00–3:00 AM. The child will often be better from warmth in general. The child will want company and may be worried about ever getting better. If there is nausea and vomiting, they will often happen at the same time and the child will be very weak after either.

- **Baptisia (Bapt) 30C**

    When Bapt is indicated you will likely see a hot and flushed face. There are often throbbing pains which cause the child to shift about trying to find a way to be comfortable. The child may find it hard to concentrate and act drugged and dopey. The child's face may look puffy and swollen with heavy eyes. The throat can be very swollen and red, and, yet, is not painful. These children are usually very thirsty.

- **Belladonna (Bell) 30C**

    As with most cases that call for Bell, you will see sudden and rapid developing symptoms. The flu starts suddenly with a hot flushed face, flushed and red skin elsewhere and glazed eyes with dilated pupils. The child may complain of pulsing or throbbing pains all over, throbbing headache, throbbing muscle pain and all are worse with motion, jarring (e.g. a bumpy car ride) or being bumped or jostled. They often have a hot head and / or body with cold hands and feet. They are

over-sensitive to light, being touched and noise. Symptoms are
generally worse at 3 PM. They are not very thirsty. There may
be sudden nausea or diarrhea.

◆ Bryonia (Bry) 30C

Bry usually covers a child who is hot, has very dry mucous
membranes and feels pain all over the body. Everything is
worse from movement of any kind and better from pressure
and being completely still. When there is a headache, it is
worse with each cough. Because movement hurts, the child
may hold the head or chest when coughing. There is great
thirst for large quantities of liquids which will be gulped down
in large quantities. The child is typically irritable and wants to
be left alone.

◆ Dulcamara (Dulc) 30C

In Dulc, the eyes are red, the throat and muscles are sore
and the cough hurts because of the muscular soreness. This
child is typically worse from cold and damp weather. Like in
Bry, there is a dryness of all the mucous membranes. You can
tell this remedy apart from Bry, however, in that most of the
symptoms are worse when the child is at rest and better when
moving about. The symptoms of Dulc are typically worse in
the evening.

◆ Eupatorium perfoliatum (Eup-per) 30C

The child will complains of soreness –a deep, hard aching
in the bones which almost feels as if the bones are broken.
There is great thirst for cold drinks or cold food which can
be vomited shortly after being consumed, as is seen in Phos.
There is a painful cough and the eyeballs hurt. Often, you will
see a chill before the fever, especially from 7–9 AM. The child
is worse with movement.

◆ Gelsemium sempervirens (Gels) 30C

The child needing Gels will often appear dull, listless, drowsy
and apathetic. There will be chills that run up and down the
back. The child may say thee body and limbs feel heavy and
weak and that the eyes feel heavy. Keeping the eyes open may
be difficult. A child needing this remedy is generally not very

thirsty. There will likely be complaints of a dull headache, especially at the back of the head and, interestingly, the headache may be better after urinating. There can also be some stiffness of the neck.

- ◆ **Mercurius solubilis (Merc) 30C**

  The child who needs Merc will not have dryness as a symptom. The child will often be very thirsty even without having a dry mouth. There is a chilliness that seems to creep along the body when symptoms begin. The breath is often foul smelling and any discharges can be thick, smelly and green. The child may be very sweaty and the symptoms are usually worse at night. The throat may be very painful.

- ◆ **Nux vomica (Nux-v) 30C**

  A child needing Nux will typically be very chilly and sensitive to cold, especially to drafts of cold air. The child will want to be all bundled up and the symptoms are worse when uncovered. The child will be cranky, irritable and very sensitive to light, smells and sounds. Like Ars, the nose can be blocked with a runny discharge at the same time. Symptoms are frequently accompanied by nausea and vomit that is very sour.

- ◆ **Phosphorus (Phos) 30C**

  The symptoms appear to move quickly and go to the chest. The child has a strong desire for large quantities of cold drinks, however, vomit may happen shortly after drinking or eating. Often, there is diarrhea that is like a gushing fire-hydrant. The child wants the company of another person and is much worse when left alone. The child will want to be held and comforted. There may be a burning sensation present when coughing.

- ◆ **Pyrogenium (Pyrog) 30C**

  This is a flu with rapidly changing and a high fever. The child is very restless during the fever. They ache all over and may complain the bed feels too hard. There is often a rapid pulse with a low temperature or a high temperature with a slow pulse.

- ◆ **Rhus toxicodendron (Rhus-t) 30C**

This child cannot get comfortable and has to frequently change position which only brings temporary relief. Muscles and joints are stiff which are worse with rest and initial movement and better with continued motion. This can be compared to a rusty gate hinge. It takes about a minute to loosen up but once moving is better. The child will be thirsty and is better from warmth, a warm bath, warm fire and worse in the cold. The child is generally worse at night and very restless.

◆ **Sulphur (Sulph) 30C**

For somone in which the flu has lingered for a long time. The child may feel hot and sweaty, run a low fever and have reddish mucous membranes. Any symptom, whether digestive or respiratory will often have a hot or burning quality. In general, any kind of heat worsens the symptoms in someone who needs Sulph.

Other Therapies

The following therapies can be used to support healing from this condition.

◆ Magnesium/Epsom Salt bath to support immune function, soothe aching muscles.

◆ Saltwater and colloidal silver gargle: two years or older (must be able to gargle) to help reduce inflammation and infection.

◆ Dry skin brushing is important with the flu to move the lymph.

◆ Lavender oil and olive oil (or coconut oil) massage reduces pain, inflammation and spasm. It can help make a child more comfortable.

1 Centers for Disease Control and Prevention. "Influenza (Flu) Flu Symptoms & Complications." cdc.gov. https://www.cdc.gov/flu/consumer/symptoms.htm (accessed February 1, 2017).

2 Ibid

3 Centers for Disease Control and Prevention. "Summary of the 2015-2016 Influenza Season." cdc.gov. https://www.cdc.gov/flu/about/season/flu-season-2015-2016.htm (accessed February 1, 2017).

4 Swamy MK, MS Akhtar, and UR Sinniah. 2016. "Antimicrobial Properties of Plant Essential Oils against Human Pathogens and Their Mode of Action: An Updated Review". Evidence-Based Complementary and Alternative Medicine : ECAM. 2016.

5 Price, Shirley, and Len Price. 2015. *Aromatherapy for health professionals.* Edinburgh [etc.]: Churchill Livingstone. 90-91

6 Papp, Rosemarie, Gert Schuback, Elmar Beck, Georg Burkard, Jürgen Bengel, Siergfried Lehrl, and Philippe Belon. 1998. "Oscillococcinum R in patients with influenza-like syndromes: A placebo-controlled double-blind evaluation". *British Homoeopathic Journal.* 87 (2): 69-76.

7 Ferley, J. "A controlled evaluation of a homoeopathic preparation in the treatment of influenza-like syndromes." *British Journal of Clinical Pharmacology.* 27 (1989): 335.

Chapter 11:
Hepatitis A

Hepatitis A is a non-enveloped RNA virus grouped as a picornavirus. It is a self-limiting, acute viral infection usually lasting less than two months but occasionally relapsing for up to six months. It is transmitted by the fecal-oral route (as when changing a dirty diaper of an infected child or touching surfaces where feces is present). The people at risk of coming into contact with hepatitis A are children living in areas with high rates of hepatitis A and consuming contaminated food and water.

There are no known long term risks or complications from infection with hepatitis A. It does not become chronic hepatitis and IgG antibodies to hepatitis A virus provide lifelong protection against the disease. In 2015, there were 1,390 cases reported in the US.[1]

This can be a hard diagnosis to make without testing. Typically, a hepatitis A diagnosis must be confirmed by a positive test for immunoglobulin M (IgM) antibody to hepatitis A virus or the person has clinical symptoms AND an exposure to a person who has laboratory-confirmed hepatitis A.

Oftentimes, there are no symptoms but signs like stomach pains, fever, nausea, abdominal pain, loss of appetite, vomiting, dark urine, clay colored stool, joint pain, jaundice or fatigue can be present. A majority of children that are less than six years old (70%) are usually asymptomatic and do not have jaundice.[2]

There are currently no conventional medical treatments available for hepatitis A.

Vitalistic Naturopathic Approach

Basic naturopathic support includes bed rest, broths, oxymel, vitamin A, C and D, zinc, ginger tea, probiotics, garlic or magic socks, medicinal baths, hydrotherapy, dry skin brushing, lymphatic massage, steam inhalation, mushrooms and NAC. If you haven't already reviewed Part 3, that is the section where we discuss these therapies at length. The following suggestions are specific for working with hepatitis.

Herbs

- Liver supporting herbs like milk thistle (*Silybum marianum*) and artichoke (*Cynara scolymus*), as a glycerite, promote liver detoxification and are liver protective.

- Herbs to use with acute or chronic hepatitis are *Bupleurum falcatum* and chanca piedra (*Phyllanthus niruri*). They are best taken as glycerites which help support and heal the liver.

- Antiviral herbs (viral meningitis) such as elderberry (*Sambucus nigra*), astragalus (*Astragalus membranaceus*), echinacea (*Echinacea angustifolia* and/or *Echinacea purpurea*), osha (*Ligusticum porteri*) can be consumed as glycerites.

- Cleavers (*Galium aparine*) as a glycerite promotes lymphatic drainage.

- Cashew milk with turmeric and raw honey to reduce inflammation.

Supplements

- Selenium, as a powder in liquid or in food, to correct selenium deficiency which can decrease the severity of hepatitis A.

- Green tea (*Camellia sinensis*) for antioxidant support (to be used during the day as it is a stimulant).

- Vitamin E (mixed tocopherols) oil squeezed out of a softgel, or as a chewable, decreases viral load.

Essential Oils

Many essential oils are toxic to the liver. Aromatherapists theorize that the early human omnivorous diet exposed us to many plants and their naturally occurring essential oils. These volatile oils, toxic to the liver in even small quantities, prompted the liver to develop more complex, broad-based detoxification pathways than are found among carnivorous mammals that eat only meat.

Because hepatitis A is an acute liver infection, you must carefully choose essential oils that support the liver and do not increase the liver's detoxification work.

The three most important essential oils to focus on while treating hepatitis A infection:

- *Ravensara aromatica* is strongly antiviral.[3]

- Bay Laurel (*Laurus nobilis*) acts as an antibacterial, antifungal, antiviral, mucolytic and expectorant.

- Greenland Moss (*Ledum groenlandicum*) stimulates regeneration of liver cells and detoxifies the liver and kidneys.[4]

Add one of the following additional oils, rotating each week:

- Carrot (*Daucus carrota*) essential oil is made from carrot seed. It is a general tonic that is restorative for liver cells and lowers high cholesterol (a function mediated by the liver).[5]

- Niaouli (*Melaleuca quinquenervia viridiflora*) acts as an antibacterial and antiviral and is traditionally used for viral hepatitis.[6]

- Thyme (*Thymus vulgaris*) thuyanol has antiviral and antibacterial effects and is an immune stimulant. It is traditionally used for viral hepatitis.

- Exotic basil oil (*Ocimum basilicum*)[7] has antimicrobial effects.

- Clove (*Eugenia caryophallata*) for viral hepatitis.[8]

- Cumin (*Cumin cyminum*)[9] aids with detoxification.

- Peppermint (*Mentha piperita*)[10] is antiviral, stimulates blood circulation through the liver, eases nausea, acts as a liver tonic and boosts immune function.

- Pimento, commonly known as allspice (*Pimenta dioicea*)[11], has antioxidant actions and is a liver tonic.

- Rosemary (*Rosmarinus officinalis*)[12] heals and detoxifies the liver, regulates bile production and enhances overall immune function.

For external use

- Chest/Foot Rub: Choose three oils to dilute in pure, organic vegetable oil. Rotate the oils you use each week, to minimize the possibility of becoming sensitized to a particular oil, which in turn potentially can sensitize you to the entire class of essential oils. Always include at least one of the following potent antiviral essential oils in your weekly blend:

- *Ravensara aromatica*

- Greenland Moss (*Ledum groenlandicu*)

- Niaouli (*Melaleuca quinquenervia viridiflora*)

Homeopathy

Up to 70% of children less than five years old with hepatitis A will often have no symptoms. If they do, it might be stomach pains, fever, nausea, abdominal pain, loss of appetite, vomiting, dark urine, clay colored stool, joint pain, jaundice or fatigue. The remedies listed here describe additional unique symptoms your child may have.

The easiest way to choose the remedy you think may work is to compare the list of symptoms you have made for your child to those listed under each remedy. Pick the one that seems to be the best match. For more explanation on how to create a list of symptoms, refer to the homeopathy section in Part 2 of this book.

The following remedies are the most common for this condition but keep in mind that the best remedy for your child may not be listed here. If you're having difficulty choosing a remedy, consider working with a homeopathic or naturopathic doctor to choose the best remedy.

- **Hepatitis A:**

   Used in the homeopathic prophylactic protocol to help reduce the risk and severity of symptoms.

- **Aurum muriaticum (Aur-m) 30C**

   There is a significant mental emotional element to this remedy. The child may imagine they have all sorts of diseases which cause palpitations of the heart. They can be very sad, depressed or irritable. There is a constant sensation of burning, stitching and tension over the area of the liver. The liver may be enlarged, swollen and tender. The spleen may also be enlarged. The abdomen is sensitive to touch and there may be a buildup of fluid in the abdominal tissues (ascites).

✦ Bryonia alba (Bry) 30C

Bry covers liver problems accompanied by rheumatic symptoms during hot or cold damp weather. There are burning pains in the liver region. The digestion is disturbed with frequent constipation and the stools are hard and dry. The great characteristics of this remedy for treating the liver are stitching and tearing pains which are worse at night and from the slightest motion. The pains are better when they are still and at rest. Typically, there is an increased thirst present.

✦ Carduus marianus (Card-m) 30C

Usually there is a dizziness or loss of balance present with a sense of heaviness and dullness over the eyes and in the temples. There is bloating of the abdomen with an increase in gas. There may be nausea and painful vomiting of a sour fluid. The liver is swollen, painful and sensitive to the touch, especially in the left lobe (more sensitive towards the center of the body than on the right side). The urine may contain bile and, if it does, will look much darker than normal. The stools may be hard, brown and knotted, soft, thin and yellow or a light gray color. There may be asthmatic symptoms along with liver symptoms. There is a sense of sadness or depression with this remedy.

✦ Chelidonium majus (Chel) 30C

Chel is a great liver remedy. Often, there are stitching pains in the liver that extend through the body to the right scapula. There is a headache that comes and goes. It begins in the back of the head at the base of skull and passes along the right side of the head to the right eye. There is frequently nausea but rarely vomiting. The child may complain of a bad (bitter) taste in the mouth and the tongue may look pointed and narrow. They may ask for and be better from drinking milk. Typically, the child has no appetite but their symptoms often improve temporarily after eating.

✦ Chionanthus virginica (Chion) 30C

In this remedy, we often see a dull headache in the forehead and the head feels full and heavy. There is an unhealthy yellow or pale brown complexion and a yellowing of the whites of the eyes. The child has little to no appetite. There is often increased saliva, sour burping and rumbling in the abdomen. There is a shooting, griping sensation in the abdomen. The urine is dark in color because it contains bile. The child is listless, apathetic and indifferent to what is going on around them.

◆ Eupatorium perfoliatum (Eup-per) 30C

Eup covers liver congestion with great soreness and painfulness of the whole body and the extremities, as if the parts had been bruised or beaten. There is a sensation of tightness, fullness and soreness in the liver. There may be a cough with soreness in the bronchi. The tongue is often coated yellow. They will vomit bile.

◆ Iris versicolor (Iris) 30C

In Iris, the liver issues are frequently accompanied by violent headaches. This may be a dull heavy headache in the forehead with nausea, or one with shooting pains in the temples with nausea and vomiting. The headache may appear with marked regularity and is preceded by blurry vision. The headache is aggravated by rest and better by continued motion which is an odd symptom as people with a headache usually want to be still. There is a loss of appetite with vomiting of a sour bitter fluid. There is painfulness in the liver and pain above the hips. The urine is dark red. The stools are soft, contain an excess of mucus, and there is a burning sensation in the anus as they pass stool.

◆ Leptandra virginica (Lept) 30C

There are frequently many liver symptoms with Lept including a dull aching in the umbilical region and pain in the right shoulder and arm. There is pain in the region of the liver which extends to the spine, and in the gall bladder which extends to the umbilical region. The child may complain of "hot" pain in the liver. There is often great rumbling in the abdomen. There may be a burning and aching in the region of the gall bladder, chilliness along the spine and an urging to have a bowel movement. The stools are tarry black with a sensation of great weakness in the abdomen after passing stool. The stool may also be profuse, black, foul smelling, soft or watery. There may be a constant dull frontal headache which extends to the temples. The tongue is coated yellow in the center and there is a bitter taste in the mouth. Jaundice may be present to some degree.

◆ Lycopodium clavatum (Lyc) 30C

Often, when Lyc is a good remedy choice, you will recognize it by an excessive accumulation of gas. The appetite is good but after a few mouthfuls the child says they are full. Then they are hungry again just a short while later. The liver is firm and sensitive to pressure. There is an aching and swelling of the lower extremities.

◆ Mercurius solubilis (Merc) 30C

In this remedy, there is great sensitivity of the liver region. The liver is enlarged and hard. There is usually some degree of jaundice. The tongue is moist and looks like it has a yellow fur. There may be a bitter or metallic taste in the mouth. There are sticking pains in the area of the liver which are worse when the child is lying on the right side. The stools are dark green and may look fatty or frothy. It is painful for them to pass stool in that it burns or hurts the tissue as they pass out of the body. The child may strain before or during passing stool and may cry out because it hurts. Their sweat and other excretions may smell bad.

◆ Nux vomica (Nux-v) 30C

In Nux-v, the stomach is sensitive to pressure about 30 minutes after each meal. Pains develop in the stomach and radiate in various directions. The liver is enlarged and tender with sticking pains. They can be very constipated with a constant urge to have a bowel movement. They may talk incessantly about having to go to the bathroom but do not feel better or fully empty after they go. The child may be very irritable and sounds, light and smells make their symptoms worse. They have painful burping which taste bitter and sour. There is nausea with a feeling that if they could only vomit, it would help them feel better. They are usually chilly and avoid drafts of air, especially cold drafts. They may crave spicy foods.

◆ A number of additional remedies should be considered

based on symptom picture and include: Arn., Aur., Bell., Carc., Crot-h., Lach., Lact., Mag-m., Nat-c., Nat-m., Nat-s., Nit-ac., Phos., Podo., Psor., Ptel., Ran-s., Sel.,Sep, Sil., Sulph., Tub.

Other Therapies

The following therapies can be used to support healing from this condition.

- Castor oil (*Ricinus communis*) pack over the liver to increase circulation and aid in toxin removal.

- Lymphatic massage to move the lymph and remove waste.

1 Centers for Disease Control and Prevention. "Viral Hepatitis Surveillance for Viral Hepatitis – United States, 2015." cdc.gov. https://www.cdc.gov/hepatitis/statistics/2015surveillance/index.htm#tabs-4-1 (accessed February 1, 2017).

2 Centers for Disease Control and Prevention. "Viral Hepatitis Hepatitis A Questions and Answers for Health Professionals." cdc.gov. https://www.cdc.gov/hepatitis/hav/havfaq.htm#general (accessed February 1, 2017).

3 Schnaubelt, Kurt. 1998. *Advanced aromatherapy: the science of essential oil therapy*. Rochester, Vt: Healing Arts Press. 86

4 Schnaubelt, Kurt. 1998. *Advanced aromatherapy: the science of essential oil therapy*. Rochester, Vt: Healing Arts Press. 72

5 Schnaubelt, Kurt. 1998. *Advanced aromatherapy: the science of essential oil therapy*. Rochester, Vt: Healing Arts Press. 62

6 Price, Shirley, and Len Price. 2015. *Aromatherapy for health professionals*. Edinburgh [etc.]: Churchill Livingstone. 90-91

7 Schnaubelt, Kurt. 1998. *Advanced aromatherapy: the science of essential oil therapy*. Rochester, Vt: Healing Arts Press. 60

8 Schnaubelt, Kurt. 1998. *Advanced aromatherapy: the science of essential oil therapy*. Rochester, Vt: Healing Arts Press. 65

9 Price, Shirley, and Len Price. 2015. *Aromatherapy for health professionals*. Edinburgh [etc.]: Churchill Livingstone. 90-91

10 Ibid

11 Ibid

12 Ibid

Chapter 12:
Hepatitis B

Hepatitis B is a virus that infects the liver. In 2015, 3370 cases were reported in the US.[1] It is transmitted from mother to child during vaginal delivery if the mother is hepatitis B positive (this is checked for all women at the beginning of pregnancy), via IV drug use or contact with the blood, saliva, semen or open wound of an infected person. Symptoms of hepatitis B include nausea, vomiting, loss of appetite, abdominal pain, fever, dark urine, clay colored stools, fatigue, joint pain and jaundice. Children less than five years old will not display any symptoms.[2] This is not a common early childhood illness.

Hepatitis B infection is concerning because it is a lifelong infection once acquired. Symptoms show up anywhere from 2–5 months after infection. People with chronic hepatitis B infection either display no symptoms or can have conditions like liver cirrhosis or liver cancer later in life. People who are most at risk of contracting hepatitis B are people engaging in risky behaviors such as unprotected sexual intercourse and IV drug use.

There are no conventional medical treatments available for acute hepatitis B. Once it becomes chronic and liver problems have developed, there are various medications used based on the type of liver disease that has manifested for the person.

Vitalistic Naturopathic Approach

Basic naturopathic support includes bed rest, broths, oxymel, vitamin A, C and D, zinc, ginger tea, probiotics, garlic or magic socks, medicinal baths, hydrotherapy, dry skin brushing, lymphatic massage, steam inhalation, mushrooms and NAC. If you haven't already reviewed Part 3, that is the section where we discuss these therapies at length. The following suggestions are specific for working with hepatitis.

Herbs

- Liver supporting herbs like milk thistle (*Silybum marianum*) and artichoke (*Cynara scolymus*), as a glycerite, promote liver detoxification and are liver protective.

- Herbs to use with acute or chronic hepatitis are *Bupleurum falcatum* and chanca piedra (*Phyllanthus niruri*). They are best taken as glycerites which help support and heal the liver.

♦ Antiviral herbs (viral meningitis) such as elderberry (*Sambucus nigra*), astragalus (*Astragalus membranaceus*), echinacea (*Echinacea angustifolia* and/or *Echinacea purpurea*), osha (*Ligusticum porteri*) can be consumed as glycerites.

♦ Cleavers (*Galium aparine*) as a glycerite promotes lymphatic drainage.

♦ Cashew milk with turmeric and raw honey to reduce inflammation.

Supplements

♦ Selenium, as a powder in liquid or in food, corrects selenium deficiency which can decrease the severity of hepatitis A.

♦ Green tea (*Camellia sinensis*) for antioxidant support (to be used during the day as it is a stimulant).

♦ Vitamin E (*mixed tocopherols*) oil squeezed out of a softgel or as a chewable decreases viral load.

Essential Oils

Many essential oils are toxic to the liver. In fact, aromatherapists theorize that the early human omnivorous diet exposed us to many plants and their naturally occurring essential oils. These volatile oils, toxic to the liver in even small quantities, prompted the liver to develop more complex, broad-based detoxification pathways than are found among carnivorous mammals that eat only meat.

Because hepatitis B is a chronic liver infection, you must carefully choose essential oils that support the liver and do not increase the liver's detoxification work. Thankfully, research provides guidance about essential oils that support liver regeneration and address the underlying infection without further stressing the liver.[3, 4] This essential oil combination was studied with persons undergoing conventional therapy (interferon and ribavirin) as well as those who chose only natural therapies. The protocol used in this study included taking essential oils internally, so you must work with a healthcare provider with advanced training in essential oils to follow this protocol. If you do not have a healthcare provider to work with, use these oils externally.

The three most important essential oils to focus on while treating hepatitis B infection:

- *Ravensara aromatica* is strongly antiviral.[5]

- Bay Laurel (*Laurus nobilis*) acts as an antibacterial, antifungal, antiviral, mucolytic and expectorant.

- Greenland Moss (*Ledum groenlandicum*) stimulates regeneration of liver cells and detoxifies the liver and kidneys.[6]

Add one of the following additional oils, rotating each week.

- Carrot (*Daucus carrota*) the essential oil is made from carrot seed. It is a general tonic that is restorative for liver cells and lowers high cholesterol (a function mediated by the liver).[7]

- Niaouli (*Melaleuca quinquenervia viridiflora*) acts as an antibacterial and antiviral and is traditionally used for viral hepatitis.[8]

- Thyme (*Thymus vulgaris*) thuyanol has antiviral and antibacterial effects and is an immune stimulant. It is traditionally used for viral hepatitis.

- Exotic basil oil (*Ocimum basilicum*)[9] has antimicrobial effects.

- Clove (*Eugenia caryophallata*) for viral hepatitis.[10]

- Cumin (*Cumin cyminum*)[11] aids with detoxification.

- Peppermint (*Mentha piperita*)[12] is antiviral, stimulates blood circulation through the liver, eases nausea, acts as a liver tonic and boosts immune function.

- Pimento, commonly known as allspice (*Pimenta dioicea*),[13] has antioxidant actions and is a liver tonic.

- Rosemary (*Rosmarinus officinalis*)[14] heals and detoxifies the liver, regulates bile production and enhances overall immune function.

Homeopathy

Most children less than five years old with hepatitis B do not have any symptoms and, in fact, this is a very rare condition in children of this age. If symptoms are present, they may include nausea, vomiting, loss of appetite, abdominal pain, fever, dark urine, clay colored stools, fatigue, joint pain and jaundice. The remedies listed here describe additional unique symptoms your child may have.

The easiest way to choose the remedy you think may work is to compare the list of symptoms you have made for your child to those listed under each remedy. Pick the one that seems to be the best match. For more explanation on how to create a list of symptoms, refer to the homeopathy section in Part 2 of this book.

The following remedies are the most common for this condition but keep in mind that the best remedy for your child may not be listed here. If you're having difficulty choosing a remedy, consider working with a homeopathic or naturopathic doctor to choose the best remedy.

- **Aurum muriaticum (Aur-m) 30C**

  There is a significant mental-emotional element to this remedy. The child may imagine they have all sorts of diseases which cause palpitations of the heart. They can be very sad, depressed or irritable. There is a constant sensation of burning, stitching and tension over the area of the liver. The liver may be enlarged, swollen and tender. The spleen may also be enlarged. The abdomen is sensitive to touch and there may be a build-up of fluid in the abdominal tissues (ascites).

- **Bryonia alba (Bry) 30C**

  Bry covers liver problems accompanied by rheumatic symptoms during hot or cold damp weather. There are burning pains in the liver region. The digestion is disturbed with frequent constipation and the stools are hard and dry. The great characteristics of this remedy for treating the liver are stitching and tearing pains which are worse at night and from the slightest motion. The pains are better when they are still and at rest. Typically, there is increased thirst present.

◆ **Carduus marianus (Card-m) 30C**

Usually there is dizziness or loss of balance present with
a sense of heaviness and dullness over the eyes and in the
temples. There is bloating of the abdomen with an increase in
gas. There may be nausea and painful vomiting of a sour fluid.
The liver is swollen, painful and sensitive to touch, especially
in the left lobe (more sensitive towards the center of the body
than on the right side). The urine may contain bile and, if it
does, will look much darker than normal. The stools may be
hard, brown and knotted, soft, thin and yellow or a light gray
color. There may be asthmatic symptoms along with liver
symptoms. There is a sense of sadness or depression with this
remedy.

◆ **Chelidonium majus (Chel) 30C**

Chel is a great liver remedy. Often, there are stitching pains
in the liver that extend through the body to the right scapula.
There is a headache that comes and goes. It begins in the back
of the head at the base of skull and passes along the right side
of the head to the right eye. There is frequently nausea but
rarely vomiting. The child may complain of a bad (bitter) taste
in the mouth and the tongue may look pointed and narrow.
They may ask for and be better from drinking milk. Typically
the child has no appetite but their symptoms often improve
temporarily after eating.

◆ **Chionanthus virginica (Chion) 30C**

In this remedy we often see a dull headache in the forehead
and the head feels full and heavy. There is an unhealthy yellow
or pale brown complexion and a yellowing of the whites of the
eyes. The child has little to no appetite. There is often increased
saliva, sour burping and rumbling in the abdomen. There is a
shooting, griping sensation in the abdomen. The urine is dark
in color because it contains bile. The child is listless, apathetic
and indifferent to what is going on around them.

◆ **Eupatorium perfoliatum (Eup-per) 30C**

Eup covers liver congestion with great soreness and painfulness
of the whole body and the extremities, as if the parts had been
bruised or beaten. There is a sensation of tightness, fullness

and soreness in the liver. There may be a cough with soreness in the bronchi. The tongue is often coated yellow and they will vomit bile.

+ **Iris versicolor (Iris) 30C**

   In Iris, the liver issues are frequently accompanied by violent headaches. This may be a dull heavy headache in the forehead with nausea or one with shooting pains in the temples with nausea and vomiting. The headache may appear with marked regularity and is preceded by blurry vision. The headache is aggravated by rest and better by continued motion which is an odd symptom as people with a headache usually want to be still. There is loss of the appetite with vomiting of a sour bitter fluid. There is painfulness in the liver and pain above the hips. The urine is dark red. The stools are soft, contain an excess of mucus, and there is a burning sensation in the anus as they pass stool.

+ **Leptandra virginica (Lept) 30C**

   There are frequently many liver symptoms with Lept including a dull aching in the umbilical region and pain in the right shoulder and arm. There is pain in the region of the liver which extends to the spine, and in the gall bladder which extends to the umbilical region. The child may complain of "hot" pain in the liver. There is often great rumbling in the abdomen. There may be a burning and aching in the region of the gall bladder, chilliness along the spine and an urging to have a bowel movement. The stools are tarry black with a sensation of great weakness in the abdomen after passing stool. The stool may also be profuse, black, foul smelling, soft or watery. There may be a constant dull frontal headache which extends to the temples. The tongue is coated yellow in the center and there is a bitter taste in the mouth. Jaundice may be present to some degree.

+ **Lycopodium clavatum (Lyc) 30C**

   Often, when Lyc is a good remedy choice, you will recognize it by an excessive accumulation of gas. The appetite is good but after a few mouthfuls the child says they are full. Then they are hungry again just a short while later. The liver is firm and sensitive to pressure. There is an aching and swelling of the lower extremities.

◆ Mercurius solubilis (Merc) 30C

In this remedy, there is great sensitivity of the liver region. The liver is enlarged and hard. There is usually some degree of jaundice. The tongue is moist and looks like it has a yellow fur. There may be a bitter or metallic taste in the mouth. There are sticking pains in the area of the liver which are worse when the child is lying on the right side. The stools are dark green and may look fatty or frothy. It is painful for them to pass stool in that it burns or hurts the tissue as they pass out of the body. The child may strain before or during passing stool and may cry out because it hurts. Their sweat and other excretions may smell bad.

◆ Nux vomica (Nux-v) 30C

In Nux-v, the stomach is sensitive to pressure about thirty minutes after each meal. Pains develop in the stomach and radiate in various directions. The liver is enlarged and tender with sticking pains. They can be very constipated with a constant urge to have a bowel movement. They may talk incessantly about having to go to the bathroom but do not feel better or fully empty after they go. The child may be very irritable and sounds, light and smells make their symptoms worse. They have painful burping which taste bitter and sour. There is nausea with a feeling that if they could only vomit it would help them feel better. They are usually chilly and avoid drafts of air, especially cold drafts. They may crave spicy foods.

- ◆ A number of additional remedies should be considered based on symptom picture and include: Arn., Aur., Bell., Carc., Crot-h., Lach., Lact., Mag-m., Nat-c., Nat-m., Nat-s., Nit-ac., Phos., Podo., Psor., Ptel., Ran-s., Sel.,Sep, Sil., Sulph., Tub.

Other Therapies

The following therapies can be used to support healing from this condition.

- Castor oil (*Ricinus communis*) pack over the liver to increase circulation and aid in toxin removal.

- Lymphatic massage to move the lymph and remove waste.

1 Centers for Disease Control and Prevention. "Surveillance for Viral Hepatitis – United States, 2015." cdc.gov. https://www.cdc.gov/hepatitis/statistics/2015surveillance/index.htm#tabs-4-1 (accessed February 1, 2017).

2 Centers for Disease Control and Prevention. "Hepatitis B FAQs for Health Professionals." cdc.gov. https://www.cdc.gov/hepatitis/hbv/hbvfaq.htm#treatment (accessed February 1, 2017).

3 GIRAUDROBERT, A. 2005. "The role of aromatherapy in the treatment of viral hepatitis". *International Journal of Aromatherapy.* 15 (4): 183-192.

4 Schnaubelt, Kurt. 2011. *The healing intelligence of essential oils: the science of advanced aromatherapy.* Rochester, Vt: Healing Arts Press. 196-203

5 Schnaubelt, Kurt. 1998. *Advanced aromatherapy: the science of essential oil therapy.* Rochester, Vt: Healing Arts Press. 86

6 Schnaubelt, Kurt. 1998. *Advanced aromatherapy: the science of essential oil therapy.* Rochester, Vt: Healing Arts Press. 72

7 Schnaubelt, Kurt. 1998. *Advanced aromatherapy: the science of essential oil therapy.* Rochester, Vt: Healing Arts Press. 62

8 Price, Shirley, and Len Price. 2015. *Aromatherapy for health professionals.* Edinburgh [etc.]: Churchill Livingstone. 90-91

9 Schnaubelt, Kurt. 1998. *Advanced aromatherapy: the science of essential oil therapy.* Rochester, Vt: Healing Arts Press. 60

10 Schnaubelt, Kurt. 1998. *Advanced aromatherapy: the science of essential oil therapy.* Rochester, Vt: Healing Arts Press. 65

11 Price, Shirley, and Len Price. 2015. *Aromatherapy for health professionals.* Edinburgh [etc.]: Churchill Livingstone. 90-91

12 Ibid

13 Ibid

14 Ibid

Chapter 13:
Hib (Haemophilus Influenzae type B)

The seasonal flu people hear about every year is a virus that mutates year after year. *Haemophilus influenzae* (Hib) is different. This is caused by a bacteria that is a normal resident of mucous membranes such as the respiratory tract, nasal passages and throat. Some children are carriers without symptoms (1–5% of unvaccinated children). If it overgrows in the body, it can cause ear infections in children. It is passed via coughing, sneezing or contact with contaminated respiratory secretions from an infected person. Children can get this infection and the body can clear it on its own. Although it rarely invades spinal fluid, heart, blood and lungs tissue, if it gets into these areas of the body that are usually free of microorganisms, it can lead to conditions like pneumonia, bacteremia, meningitis, or cellulitis among others.[1]

The national estimates of these types of invasive disease is 6,100 cases. According to 2015 data collected on all ages from ten states, fifty-six cases[2] of Hib infections ended in meningitis and 472 ended up in pneumonia.[3] In very rare cases, it can lead to shock, coma, seizures and death (four deaths due to meningitis and eighty-one deaths due to pneumonia with bacteremia across all ages collectively).[4]

The most recent CDC data available from 2015 showed that for children age less than one year to seventeen years old, there were three cases of Hib in the United States. This is the only type known to be contagious. Non-B and non-typeable Hib, while still serious to the infected child, do not have an increased risk of transmission.

The reason Hib is concerning to health practitioners and parents alike is because it can cause meningitis if it enters the spinal cord. Symptoms of meningitis can start out as a fever and headache, followed by sensitivity to light, mental confusion and the tell-tale sign of a stiff neck. Babies can be lethargic and irritable, have little muscle strength and may have no appetite. A child infected with Hib runs the risk of later having seizures, language delays, learning disabilities, vision loss, retardation, abscesses, anaphylaxis, joint pain, rashes, edema, blood infection and diabetes. A sudden change in alertness or severe headache in children is cause for concern. This is important to remember for any condition that can cause meningitis.

The main concern with Hib is meningitis for children that are less than one year old. Also, epiglottitis is the main concern for children that are around two years of age. For the reported number of cases, it is unknown if those children were unvaccinated or vaccinated. If they were vaccinated, we do not know how many vaccine injections they received. Mainstream medicine considers unvaccinated children to be most at risk. However, CDC data from 2010–2011 showed that of the 2500 cases of Hib infection, 36% of the 6-month yo 5-year-old children were fully vaccinated.

The incubation period is likely 2–7 days and symptoms start like the flu with fever and chills, cough, muscle aches (especially in back, arms and legs) and a headache. There can be nausea and vomiting, more common in young children, and a sore throat. If it affects the lungs, it can cause a person to have chest pains accompanied by a cough and difficulty breathing. If it affects the blood, the person can have nausea, vomiting, diarrhea, shortness of breath and mental confusion.

In the case a child is diagnosed with Hib infection, medical doctors will start antibiotics to prevent an invasive infection. Unfortunately, the bacteria is becoming resistant to first line antibiotics so an infection will require hospitalization.[5]

Vitalistic Naturopathic Approach

The most protective factor against Hib for infants and children is breastfeeding,[6] ideally for longer than three months. With every additional week of breastfeeding, the risk of contracting this disease decreases.[7] The protective effects of breastfeeding last for many years. Breastfed infants have decreased incidence for up to 5-10 years later. By five years of age, most children have normal levels of Hib colonization to produce immunity to the disease.[8]

Basic naturopathic support includes bed rest, broths, oxymel, vitamin A, C and D, zinc, ginger tea, probiotics, garlic or magic socks, medicinal baths, hydrotherapy, dry skin brushing, lymphatic massage, steam inhalation, mushrooms and NAC. If you haven't already reviewed Part 3, that is the section where we discuss these therapies at length. The following suggestions are specific for working with Haemophilus Influenzae.

Herbs

- Ginger (*Zingiber officinale*) as a tea can address nausea, vomiting and ease pain.

- Elderberry (*Sambucus nigra*) is best taken as a syrup or glycerite. It is a general immune tonic increasing white blood cell activity and has antimicrobial effects.

- Astragalus (*Astragalus membranaceus*) is best taken as a syrup or glycerite. It is an adaptogenic herb which restores normal function, has anti-inflammatory and antiviral effects and is an immunomodulator.

- Sage (*Salvia officinalis*) as a tea with raw honey and lemon or as a glycerite boosts the immune system and is drying which decreases mucus.

- Berberine containing antibacterial herbs: goldenseal (*Hydrastis canadensis*), barberry (*Berberis vulgaris*), Oregon grape root (*Mahonia aquifolium*), coptis (*Coptis chinensis*). Because of their taste, they are best consumed as glycerites. Choose one of these herbs.

- Echinacea (*Echinacea angustifolia* and/or *Echinacea purpurea*) as a tincture or glycerite is supportive to the immune system and has antimicrobial effects.

- Lomatium (*Lomatium dissectum*) used as a tea or glycerite is a strong antimicrobial (bacteria and viruses) and has an affinity for the lungs. It stimulates the production of white blood cells, is immunomodulating, enhances the production and release of mucus, and eases spasms connected to cough. It is also a nutritive that supports the body during long-standing illness.

Supplements

- Vitamin A flush: This is a treatment that can be highly effective but should be done under the supervision of a naturopathic physician or other qualified health care practitioner.

Essential Oils

Inhaling essential oils rapidly delivers healing support to the respiratory system, and through absorption in the lungs, to the entire body. For ALL essential oils: avoid using a cold diffuser that runs continuously. Long term (e.g. more than 45–60 minutes), ongoing exposure to any essential oil stresses the liver's detoxification pathways, particularly for young children. Ongoing exposures also increases the risk of sensitizing your child to that essential oil in particular and to essential oils in general. In this condition, essential oils quickly address the virus itself and provide relief for the uncomfortable symptoms. Two potent healing allies that specifically address Hib infection include:

- Russian Wormwood (*Artemesia verstita*) authentic (whole) essential oil is more effective than isolated constituents.[9]

- Spotted bee balm (*Monarda punctata*)[10]

- Another essential oil found to be effective against the H2N2 (pandemic) influenza:

- Patchouli (*Pogostemon cablin*)[11]

Chest and foot rub: choose from the essential oils listed above. Rotate the combination of essential oils you are using every 2–3 days, to avoid the skin becoming sensitized to the essential oils.

Inhalation: Choose one or a combination of the above essential oils. Test the oils first on a tissue and inhale to make sure you like the smell of the combination (if your nose is clear enough to smell!) You will have benefit from the essential oils even if you have no sense of smell. If you can smell, you will be more likely to use the inhaler if you enjoy the scent if using conventional therapies.

Homeopathy

A child with Hib may have symptoms like the flu with fever and chills, cough, muscle aches (especially in back, arms and legs) and a headache. There can be nausea and vomiting and a sore throat or chest pains accompanied by a cough and difficulty breathing. The remedies listed here describe additional unique symptoms your child may have.

The easiest way to choose the remedy you think may work is to compare the list of symptoms you have made for your child to those listed under each remedy. Pick the one that seems to be the best match. For more explanation on how to create a list of symptoms, refer to the homeopathy section in Part 2 of this book.

The following remedies are the most common for this condition but keep in mind that the best remedy for your child may not be listed here.

If you're having difficulty choosing a remedy, consider working with a homeopathic or naturopathic doctor to choose the best remedy.

Prophylactic remedies to help reduce risk (you can use any or all):

- **Haemophilus influenzae B vaccinus (Haem-i-b-vc 30C):**

   Used in the homeopathic prophylactic protocol to help reduce the risk and severity of symptoms.

- **Influenzinum 30C (current year):**

   Used in the homeopathic prophylactic protocol to help reduce the risk and severity of symptoms.

- **Oscillococcinum:**

   As a preventative at the beginning of flu season.[12, 13]

If symptoms of Hib are present:

- **Arsenicum Album (Ars) 30C**

   You will notice symptoms of chill, weakness, restlessness and anxiety. The child will be thirsty for frequent sips of cold water. Discharges from a blocked and stuffy nose will be thin and watery. The child and symptoms will be worse from cold air, cold applications and from 1–3 AM. The child will often be better from warmth in general. The child will want company and may be worried about ever getting better. If there is nausea and vomiting, they will often happen at the same time and the child will be very weak after either.

- **Baptisia (Bapt) 30C**

   When Bapt is indicated you will likely see a hot and flushed face. There are often throbbing pains which cause the child to shift about trying to find a way to be comfortable. The child may find it hard to concentrate and act drugged and dopey. The child's face may look puffy and swollen with heavy eyes. The throat can be very swollen and red, and, yet, is not painful. These children are usually very thirsty.

- **Belladonna (Bell) 30C**

As with most cases that call for Bell, you will see sudden and rapid developing symptoms. The flu starts suddenly with a hot flushed face, flushed and red skin elsewhere and glazed eyes with dilated pupils. The child may complain of pulsing or throbbing pains all over, throbbing headache, throbbing muscle pain and all are worse with motion, jarring (e.g. a bumpy car ride) or being bumped or jostled. They often have a hot head and / or body with cold hands and feet. They are over-sensitive to light, being touched and noise. Symptoms are generally worse at 3 PM. They are not very thirsty. There may be sudden nausea or diarrhea.

♦ **Bryonia (Bry) 30C**

Bry usually covers a child who is hot, has very dry mucous membranes and feels pain all over the body. Everything is worse from movement of any kind and better from pressure and being completely still. When there is a headache, it is worse with each cough. Because movement hurts, the child may hold the head or chest when coughing. There is great thirst for large quantities of liquids which will be gulped down in large quantities. The child is typically irritable and wants to be left alone.

♦ **Dulcamara (Dulc) 30C**

In Dulc, the eyes are red, the throat and muscles are sore and the cough hurts because of the muscular soreness. This child is typically worse from cold and damp weather. Like in Bry, there is a dryness of all the mucous membranes. You can tell this remedy apart from Bry, however, in that most of the symptoms are worse when the child is at rest and better when moving about. The symptoms of Dulc are typically worse in the evening.

♦ **Eupatorium perfoliatum (Eup-per) 30C**

The child will complains of soreness –a deep, hard aching in the bones which almost feels as if the bones are broken. There is great thirst for cold drinks or cold food which can be vomited shortly after being consumed, as is seen in Phos. There is a painful cough and the eyeballs hurt. Often, you will see a chill before the fever, especially from 7–9 AM. The child is worse with movement.

◆ Gelsemium sempervirens (Gels) 30C

The child needing Gels will often appear dull, listless, drowsy and apathetic. There will be chills that run up and down the back. The child may say thee body and limbs feel heavy and weak and that the eyes feel heavy. Keeping the eyes open may be difficult. A child needing this remedy is generally not very thirsty. There will likely be complaints of a dull headache, especially at the back of the head and, interestingly, the headache may be better after urinating. There can also be some stiffness of the neck.

◆ Mercurius solubilis (Merc) 30C

The child who needs Merc will not have dryness as a symptom. The child will often be very thirsty even without having a dry mouth. There is a chilliness that seems to creep along the body when symptoms begin. The breath is often foul smelling and any discharges can be thick, smelly and green. The child may be very sweaty and the symptoms are usually worse at night. The throat may be very painful.

◆ Nux vomica (Nux-v) 30C

A child needing Nux will typically be very chilly and sensitive to cold, especially to drafts of cold air. The child will want to be all bundled up and the symptoms are worse when uncovered. The child will be cranky, irritable and very sensitive to light, smells and sounds. Like Ars, the nose can be blocked with a runny discharge at the same time. Symptoms are frequently accompanied by nausea and vomit that is very sour.

◆ Phosphorus (Phos) 30C

The symptoms appear to move quickly and go to the chest. The child has a strong desire for large quantities of cold drinks, however, vomit may happen shortly after drinking or eating. Often, there is diarrhea that is like a gushing fire-hydrant. The child wants the company of another person and is much worse when left alone. The child will want to be held and comforted. There may be a burning sensation present when coughing.

- **Pyrogenium (Pyrog) 30C**

    This is a flu with rapidly changing and a high fever. The child is very restless during the fever. They ache all over and may complain the bed feels too hard. There is often a rapid pulse with a low temperature or a high temperature with a slow pulse.

- **Rhus toxicodendron (Rhus-t) 30C**

    This child cannot get comfortable and has to frequently change position which only brings temporary relief. Muscles and joints are stiff which are worse with rest and initial movement and better with continued motion. This can be compared to a rusty gate hinge. It takes about a minute to loosen up but once moving is better. The child will be thirsty and is better from warmth, a warm bath, warm fire and worse in the cold. The child is generally worse at night and very restless.

- **Sulphur (Sulph) 30C**

    For somone in which the flu has lingered for a long time. The child may feel hot and sweaty, run a low fever and have reddish mucous membranes. Any symptom, whether digestive or respiratory will often have a hot or burning quality. In general, any kind of heat worsens the symptoms in someone who needs Sulph.

Other Therapies

The following therapies can be used to support healing from this condition.

- Magnesium/Epsom Salt bath to support immune function, soothe aching muscles.

- Saltwater and colloidal silver gargle: two years or older (must be able to gargle) to help reduce inflammation and infection.

- Dry skin brushing is important with Hib to move the lymph.

- Lavender oil and olive oil (or coconut oil) massage reduces pain, inflammation and spasm. It can help make a child more comfortable.

1 Centers for Disease Control and Prevention. "Types of Haemophilus influenzae Infections." cdc.gov. https://www.cdc.gov/hi-disease/about/types-infection.html (accessed February 1, 2017).

2 Centers for Disease Control and Prevention. "ABCs Report: Haemophilus influenzae, 2015." cdc.gov. https://www.cdc.gov/abcs/reports-findings/survreports/hib15.html (accessed February 1, 2017).

3 Ibid

4 Ibid

5 Centers for Disease Control and Prevention. "Epidemiology and Prevention of Vaccine-Preventable Diseases Hacmophilus influenzae type b." cdc.gov. https://www.cdc.gov/vaccines/pubs/pinkbook/hib.html#medical (accessed February 1, 2017).

6 Centers for Disease Control and Prevention. "Epidemiology and Prevention of Vaccine-Preventable Diseases Haemophilus influenzae type b." cdc.gov. https://www.cdc.gov/vaccines/pubs/pinkbook/hib.html (accessed February 1, 2017).

7 Hanson, Lars A. 1998. "Breastfeeding Provides Passive and Likely Long-Lasting Active Immunity". Annals of Allergy, Asthma & Immunology. 81 (6): 523-537.

8 Andrews, H. and H. Zwickey. "The Vaccine Balancing Act" Seminar. 2009.

9 Yang C, DH Hu, and Y Feng. 2015. "Essential oil of Artemisia vestita exhibits potent in vitro and in vivo antibacterial activity: Investigation of the effect of oil on biofilm formation, leakage of potassium ions and survival curve measurement". *Molecular Medicine Reports*. 12 (4): 5762-70.

10 Li, Hong, Yang, Tian, Li, Fei-Yan, Yao, Yan, and Sun, Zhong-Min. 2014. *Antibacterial activity and mechanism of action of Monarda punctata essential oil and its main components against common bacterial pathogens in respiratory tract*. e-Century Publishing Corporation.

11 Swamy MK, MS Akhtar, and UR Sinniah. 2016. "Antimicrobial Properties of Plant Essential Oils against Human Pathogens and Their Mode of Action: An Updated Review". Evidence-Based Complementary and Alternative Medicine : ECAM. 2016.

12 Papp, Rosemarie, Gert Schuback, Elmar Beck, Georg Burkard, Jürgen Bengel, Siergfried Lehrl, and Philippe Belon. 1998. "Oscillococcinum R in patients with influenza-like syndromes: A placebo-controlled double-blind evaluation". *British Homoeopathic Journal*. 87 (2): 69-76.

13 Ferley, J. "A controlled evaluation of a homoeopathic preparation in the treatment of influenza-like syndromes." *British Journal of Clinical Pharmacology*. 27 (1989): 335.

Chapter 14:
HPV (Human Papillomavirus)

Human Papilloma virus (HPV) is a virus that has well over 100 strains and causes warts. Warts can show up anywhere on the body. For children, they are commonly found on the hands and feet. These kinds of warts are easily treated with a number of different natural therapies. The form of HPV most people are concerned with is the type that is sexually transmitted and causes genital warts.[1]

HPV that is sexually transmitted can have warts, but don't always. When no warts are present, the infection can resolve on its own or can be easily treated naturally. Many conventional doctors take a wait and watch approach when no warts are present. When warts appear, they can be flat, pink, red, raised, flesh-colored or have a cauliflower appearance. Warts can easily be treated. What is important to note with HPV is the type. There are low risk strains (HPV 6 and 11) that cause 90% of infections. High risk strains (HPV 16 and 18 and five others less commonly seen: 31, 33, 45, 52, 58) can lead to 70% of cervical cancer or, less commonly, cancer of the throat or mouth. Treated early, these infections can resolve and not lead to complications.[2, 3, 4]

Oftentimes, HPV infection is asymptomatic. In women and sexually active young girls, it can occasionally cause mild vaginal itching.

Currently, 79 million people are noted to have HPV. Approximately 14 million new cases are diagnosed every year. It is so common that everyone is expected to be infected with some type of it at some point in their lives.[5] The types causing genital warts are not of concern for young children and infants. It can potentially affect them once they become sexually active in their later years of life.

To date, there is no conventional medical treatment for HPV. If they are present, warts will be treated, but there is no specific antiviral medication available to treat HPV.

Vitalistic Naturopathic Approach

Basic naturopathic support includes bed rest, broths, oxymel, vitamin A, C and D, zinc, ginger tea, probiotics, garlic or magic socks, medicinal baths, hydrotherapy, dry skin brushing, lymphatic massage, steam inhalation, mushrooms and NAC. If you haven't already reviewed Part 3, that is the section where we discuss these therapies at length. The following suggestions are specific for working with HPV.

Herbs

• Green tea (*Camelia sinensis*) is a potent antioxidant (to be used during the day as it is a stimulant).

• Antiviral herbs (viral meningitis) such as elderberry (*Sambucus nigra*), astragalus (*Astragalus membranaceus*), echinacea (*Echinacea angustifolia* and/or *Echinacea purpurea*), osha (*Ligusticum porteri*) can be consumed as glycerites.

• Curcumin (*Curcuma longa*) is best as a capsule for its powerful antioxidant effects.

Supplements

• AHCC (active constituent from mushroom) is best as a powder or capsule for antiviral effects.

• Beta carotene as a capsule for immune system stimulation.

Essential Oils

A handful of essential oils, all with potent antiviral activity, have been researched and found to be effective in treating HPV.[6] These can be applied topically on the skin but not internally in the vagina:

• Cortex (*Cinnamomum verum*)

• Lime (*Citrus aurantifolia*)

• Lemon (*Citrus limon*)

• Tea tree (*Melaleuca alternifolia*) essential oil can be used as a suppository or salve that is applied vaginally. See recipe in The Apothecary section.

Homeopathy

Children with HPV usually have no symptoms. There are many kinds of HPV and all have the capacity to cause warts all over the body, including genital warts. There is not a homeopathic remedy that can be considered prophylactic. In addition, there is not a particular remedy that treats only the warts of genital HPV. However, homeopathy has been shown to be highly effective in resolving warts,[7] and therefore it is worth discussing HPV in general here as it pertains to homeopathy.

It can be complicated to treat HPV at home, and we encourage you to work with a professionally trained homeopath or naturopathic doctor to address HPV in which genital warts have manifested. The following remedies are commonly discussed in the literature and are frequently used to address warts depending on the individual case and presentation. They describe additional unique symptoms your child may have or the type of warts they may have. Here is a link to a "Quick Reference Wart Rubrics" document: https://www.vitalhealthpublishing.com/wart-rubrics.

The easiest way to choose the remedy you think may work is to compare the list of symptoms you have made for your child to those listed under each remedy. Pick the one that seems to be the best match. For more explanation on how to create a list of symptoms, refer to the homeopathy section in Part 2 of this book.

The following remedies are the most common for this condition but keep in mind that the best remedy for your child may not be listed here. If you're having difficulty choosing a remedy, consider working with a homeopathic or naturopathic doctor to choose the best remedy.

- **Antimonium crudum (Ant-c) 30C**

   Warts may look hard, smooth and often appear in groups. Warts may also look cauliflower-like or horn-like. They can be painful or painless warts. Although the warts may be anywhere, a very common area is the sole of the foot and back of the hands. Along with warts, there may be extreme sensitivity to heat, irritability and digestive issues.

- **Argentum nitricum (Arg-n) 30C**

   Warts are common on the palate or near the anus. The warts are brownish and hard to the touch and ulcerate easily. There may also be mental emotional issues (a different state than is normal) and digestive symptoms such as nausea, loss of appetite, abdominal pains or increased gas. Typically, the child does not want to be hot and is very sensitive to heat.

- **Calcarea carbonica (Calc-c) 30C**

  Many different kinds of warts can be treated with this remedy:

  - Round, hard, solitary warts

  - Warts that grow inward and have a horny wall surrounding a central depression

  - Black and fleshy, hard and horny, sometimes inflamed and painful warts

  - Round, soft at base, almost the color of skin with hard upper surface warts

  - Rough, whitish, horny warts

  The warts may itch and bleed, be inflamed, sting, have a discharge and/ or form ulcers. They may be located on the face, neck, arms, hands, male or female genitals or eyelids. The hands and feet may be clammy and there may be an overall increased level of perspiration.

- **Causticum (Caust) 30C**

  Caust warts also tend to be hard, inflamed, and painful. The skin can be whitish-yellow or appear to look "dirty" even when clean. This remedy can help old, large warts on the face (especially the nose), under the fingernails, or warts on the fingertips that bleed easily.

- **Dulcamara (Dulc) 30C**

  These warts are often soft and have a brownish to black color. They are typically located on the backs of the hands, on the face and on the back. This is a remedy to consider if the warts are accompanied by joint pains that are worse in the cold, damp or humid weather.

- **Graphites (Graph) 30C**

  The warts of Graph are typically cauliflower shaped or corn-like warts around the fingernails and toenails or on the palms or soles of the feet. They may be tinged with yellow. There may be warts present around female genitalia. There may be a sticky discharge from the wart which smells like old cheese or herring brine. The skin is dry, rough, irritable and breaks open easily with a discharge that is gluey or yellow and crusty. The child may be extremely sensitive to cold and may have various digestive issues.

◆ **Lycopodium (Lyc) 30C**

These warts may appear as single warts or in groups. Often, they are located on the face, tongue, male or female genitalia, upper arms and fingers. The warts may itch and are often large, jagged, furrowed, split and look like they have a stalk. There may be a discharge and the warts may bleed easily.

◆ **Nitricum acidum (Nit-ac) 30C**

Nit-ac warts are large, fissured or golden-yellow. They itch, sting or bleed upon washing. Often the warts may grow inward and have a horny wall surrounding a central depression. The warts appear on female genitals, anus, cervical region, inside the nose, on the external throat, sternum, eyelids and inner or outer corners of the eyes. The warts may be moist, cauliflower like, hard, fissured or cracked, large, indented or inflamed. There is a pricking pain that is worse at night. They emit a foul discharge and may bleed on touch. There can be splinter-like pains in the warts or anywhere. Touching the wart or exposing it to cold will cause pain.

◆ **Ruta graveolens (Ruta) 30C:**

Plantar warts, especially on the palms of the hand.

◆ **Sepia (Sep) 30C**

These warts are small, flat, hard, dark brown in color and often have a horny growth in the center. There is a sensation of itching in the wart. They are located on male or female genitalia, upper lips, fingers and face. The skin can be blotched, raw, rough, hard or cracked.

◆ **Thuja occidentalis (Thuj) 30C**

This is the most common remedy for many different kinds of warts. If no other remedy is obviously indicated, consider

Thuja. Warts usually occur as a single wart, not in groups. They may be jagged, smell or bleed easily. They can be broad, conical, flat, stalk-like indented or fan-shaped in appearance. They are typically reddish in color. The warts have a tendency to split from their edge or from the surface. They are usually located on the back, cervical region, upper limb, face, nose, eyebrows, eyes, eyelids and external throat. Warts on any part of body can have little necks and are called fig warts and Thuj is very good for these. There can be long warts of the same size all the way out (tubular warts). Wart-like outgrowths can appear on the back of the hand, on the chin and other places. Warts can be large, seedy and or stalk-like. They may ooze occasionally. This remedy is commonly needed for anal or genital warts. There may be other growths or tumors.

Other Therapies

The following therapies can be used to support healing from this condition.

- ◆ Vaginal suppositories with calendula, vitamin A, tea tree essential oil, green tea, marshmallow (*Althea officinalis*), vitamin E, thuja essential oil for local antiviral, antioxidant and soothing effects.

- ◆ Vaginal steaming with basil, oregano, rose and thyme to increase circulation to the vaginal area (can be used by men as well).

- ◆ Constitutional hydrotherapy for overall immune stimulation and to promote healing.

- ◆ Physiotherapy: Microcurrent electrical stimulation for regeneration of new cells.

1 Web MD. "What Is HPV??" webmd.com. http://www.webmd.com/sexual-conditions/hpv-genital-warts/hpv-virus-information-about-human-papillomavirus#1 (accessed February 1, 2017).

2 Ibid

3 Web MD. "How Do I Know If I Have HPV?" webmd.com. http://www.webmd.com/sexual-conditions/hpv-genital-warts/hpv-symptoms-tests (accessed February 1, 2017).

4 Centers for Disease Control and Prevention. "HPV and Oropharyngeal Cancer." cdc.gov. https://www.cdc.gov/cancer/hpv/basic_info/hpv_oropharyngeal.htm (accessed February 1, 2017).

5 Centers for Disease Control and Prevention. "Human Papillomavirus (HPV) Genital HPV Infection - Fact Sheet." cdc.gov. https://www.cdc.gov/std/hpv/stdfact-hpv.htm (accessed February 1, 2017).

6 Price, Shirley, and Len Price. 2015. *Aromatherapy for health professionals*. Edinburgh [etc.]: Churchill Livingstone. 90-91

7 Gupta, Ramji, O.P. Bhardwaj, and R.K. Manchanda. 1991. "Homœopathy in the treatment of warts". *British Homoeopathic Journal*. 80 (2): 108-111.

Chapter 15:
Measles (Rubeola)

Measles elimination from the Americas was achieved in 2002 and has been sustained since then, with only imported and importation-related measles cases coming from other countries that have had outbreaks like England, France, Germany, India and the Philippines.[1] The highest rates are seen in developing nations with malnutrition which is an important factor in the severity of symptoms.[2] However, in 2011, the CDC reported sixteen outbreaks of measles with 220 measles cases in the U.S. Most of them were imported cases in unvaccinated persons,[3] and from January 1st-May 20th, 2017, there were 100 U.S. cases of measles.[4]

Measles is a member of the Morbillivirus, which is part of the Paramyxoviridae family. It is a contagious illness caused by a single-stranded, enveloped RNA virus. It is transmitted via respiratory droplets that come from an infected person coughing or sneezing. Children at most risk of developing severe complications are less than five years old. With mass vaccinations, susceptible ages of infection have been pushed out to older than ten years old.

Symptoms of a measles infection include cough, runny nose, sensitivity to light, itchy rash, fever, loss of appetite, diarrhea and generalized swelling of lymph nodes in front of the ears. The most common complication of measles is diarrhea (8%) followed by ear infections (7%), and pneumonia (6%). Rare but more severe complications include hearing loss (unilateral or bilateral), encephalitis, pneumonia and degenerative disease of the central nervous system caused by persistent measles infection (occurs in 5–10 out of every million cases). Deaths are rare but can occur due to pneumonia in children younger than five years old.[5] Severity of measles is seen in malnourished children mostly in Africa.[6]

Measles typically begins with a high fever, cough, runny nose and red, watery eyes. Two or three days after those symptoms begin you may or may not see tiny white or red spots (Koplik spots) inside the mouth. These spots can be on the palate, inside the cheeks, lips or on the tongue. The typical rash of measles starts 3–5 days after the initial symptoms. These start as flat red spots along the hairline of the face which then spreads downward to the neck, trunk, arms, legs, and feet. Small raised bumps may appear on top of the flat red spots and the spots may look like they are growing together as they spread from the head to the rest of the body. The rash may itch and there may be a spike in the fever when the rash appears. The rash clears in about 7 days and the fever subsides. If treated very early with vitalistic approaches, the rash may not develop and the duration of the illness can be shortened. In addition to general support, rest and fluids, there are a number of other natural therapeutics to consider.

The only treatment available through conventional medicine for measles is high doses of Vitamin A. They do not have any specific antiviral treatment. They may suggest topical lotions or creams to relieve itching. Aspirin is contraindicated.[7]

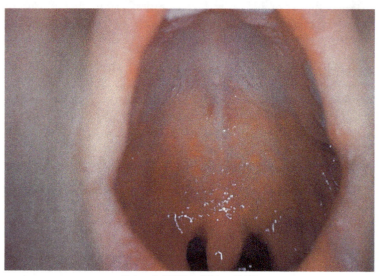

Photo credit: CDC/ Heinz F. Eichenwald, MD

Vitalistic Naturopathic Approach

Since children with measles can have sensitivity to light, it's best to have them resting in bed in a dimly lit room for children with light sensitivity. Basic naturopathic support includes bed rest, broths, oxymel, vitamin A, C and D, zinc, ginger tea, probiotics, garlic or magic socks, medicinal baths, hydrotherapy, dry skin brushing, lymphatic massage, steam inhalation, mushrooms and NAC. If you haven't already reviewed Part 3, that is the section where we discuss these therapies at length. The following suggestions are specific for working with measles.

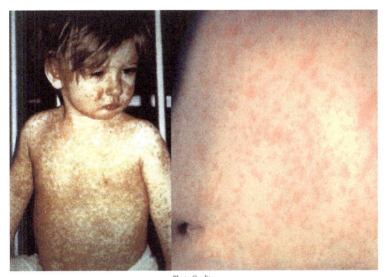

Photo Credits:
CDC/NIP/Barbara Rice - http://phil.cdc.gov/phil/ (ID#: 132), Public Domain, https://commons.wikimedia.org/w/index.php?curid=210382
CDC/ Heinz F. Eichenwald, MD

Herbs

♦ Nettles (*Urtica dioica*) as a tea or glycerite soothes itchiness.

♦ Lemon balm (*Melissa officinalis*) as a tea or glycerite acts as a mild pain reliever, has antiviral effects, eases anxiety by calming the nervous system.

♦ Burdock (*Arctium lappa*) as a tea or a base for a soup helps skin recover and heal more quickly.

♦ Antiviral herbs (viral meningitis) such as elderberry (*Sambucus nigra*), astragalus (*Astragalus membranaceus*), echinacea (*Echinacea angustifolia* and/or *Echinacea purpurea*), osha (*Ligusticum porteri*) can be consumed as glycerites.

Supplements

♦ Vitamin A flush: This is a treatment that can be highly effective, but should be done under the supervision of a naturopathic physician or other qualified health care practitioner.

Essential Oils

Essential oils can help address the underlying viral infection that causes measles as well as soothe the itching.

- Ravensara aromatica[8] has strong antiviral activity.

- German chamomile (*Matricaria chamomilla*) soothes skin irritation and itching.

- Tea tree (*Melaleuca alternifolia*) also has antiviral effects and is helpful to soothe any skin irritation.

- Lavender (*Lavandula angustifolia*) soothes the skin, reduces itching, and has mild antiviral effects. Lavender also has a calming effect which can be very helpful for children suffering with itching and other symptoms.

You can use this combination of three essential oils in the bath:

- Two drops each of ravensara, German chamomile (or lavender) and tea tree to one tablespoon of milk (cow, goat, almond, coconut, hemp, etc.) The oil and protein in the milk helps to disperse the essential oil in the bathwater. Avoid adding essential oils directly to the bathwater. They do not disperse and can cause skin irritation.

- Add to a warm bath and soak as long as desired.

- Create an oil to rub into the skin. If you are an adult applying the oil to a child's skin, use latex-free gloves to avoid contaminating yourself and others.

- Add two drops of ravensara, German chamomile, and tea tree essential oils to a tablespoon of pure, organic vegetable oil. Rub into the skin 3–4 times a day. Rub the oil first into the soles of the feet; then into the affected areas.

- For children under six years old, dilute the essential oils in two tablespoons of pure, organic vegetable oil.

Homeopathy

A child with measles will likely start with symptoms of a high fever, cough, runny nose and red, watery eyes. The typical rash of measles starts along the hairline of the face 3–5 days after the initial symptoms. The rash then spreads downward to the neck, trunk, arms, legs and feet. Small raised bumps may appear on top of the flat red spots and the spots may look like they are growing together as they spread from the head to the rest of the body. The rash may itch and there may be a spike in the fever when the rash appears.The remedies listed here describe additional unique symptoms your child may have.

The easiest way to choose the remedy you think may work is to compare the list of symptoms you have made for your child to those listed under each remedy. Pick the one that seems to be the best match. For more explanation on how to create a list of symptoms, refer to the homeopathy section in Part 2 of this book.

The following remedies are the most common for this condition but keep in mind that the best remedy for your child may not be listed here. If you're having difficulty choosing a remedy, consider working with a homeopathic or naturopathic doctor to choose the best remedy.

- **Morbillinum (Morb) 30C:**

    Used in the homeopathic prophylactic protocol to help reduce the risk and severity of symptoms.

- **Aconitum napellus (Acon) 30C**

    Acon may be useful at the beginning when the symptoms resemble that of the common cold. There may be chilliness, restlessness, dry skin and thirst especially at night. This remedy is also good when symptoms such as red eyes and sensitivity to light are present. There may be a fever with a quick full pulse and a dry barking cough. Often the child's skin is burning hot and the rash may itch.

- **Antimonium tartaricum (Ant-t) 30C**

    The rash is not well developed if it even comes out at all. What will guide you to this remedy, more than the rash is a symptom of great rattling of mucus in the chest without expectoration on coughing. You hear the rattling when they cough and you might think to yourself that if they would just do one big cough it would all come up, but it doesn't. The child has painful breathing with bluish or purplish face and drowsiness. When bronchitis or pneumonia predominates, this is a useful remedy.

+ **Apis mellifica (Apis) 30C**

The rash of measles that is best treated with Apis is one where the spots look less like spots and more like blotches as if the spots have grown together. There can be a swelling and redness to the skin and swelling of the throat. The child may have difficulty breathing and is much worse in a warm room. They are usually not thirsty, worse from heat and much better in the cool air.

+ **Arsenicum album (Ars) 30C**

There is a great deal of weakness in Ars with a poorly developed rash if there is one at all. The child may be very restless with great anxiety. Diarrhea with offensive stools can be present and is usually followed by great exhaustion. Even without a rash, there can be great itching and burning of the skin which is better from warm application and a hot bath. The symptoms are worse after midnight. The child is very thirsty for small quantities of ice cold water at frequent intervals.

+ **Belladonna (Bell) 30C**

The symptoms of Bell come on very suddenly. The child is restless and has a throbbing headache, flushed face and red eyes. Nervous symptoms predominate and they may have convulsions when the rash appears. In measles when the throat becomes sore, the child will have difficulty swallowing and may have pricking pains. You may see a high fever (103+) with an overactive brain (child is talkative and cannot settle down). There is a dry barking or spasmodic cough towards midnight and a great restlessness in that they cannot lie still.

+ **Bryonia alba (Bry) 30C**

There is often a lot of mucus and congestion present in the head, nose and throat which has a tendency to move into the bronchial system. If there is a cough, it will likely be hard and dry with tearing pains in the chest. The rash can be slow to appear but once established it is widespread but may disappear suddenly. If you see this sudden disappearance of the rash and the child appears very tired or irritable, and the rest of the symptoms match, Bry will be a good choice. In general, the child has greatly decreased energy, irritability, lack of appetite and is thirsty for large quantities of water at infrequent intervals. The child prefers to lie down quietly as slightest motion causes stitching pains in the chest. In general, movement aggravates the child needing Bry.

◆ Cuprum metallicum (Cupr) 30C

Cupr is a good remedy to consider if there are convulsions present that started after the rash cleared up. This child may wake suddenly from sleep and have a frightening convulsion with a bluish face. This is also a good remedy to consider when the measles are complicated with bronchitis, a cold clammy sweat at night and and cramps in the fingers and toes.

◆ Gelsemium sempervirens (Gels) 30C

This is a remedy to consider at the beginning of measles if the child is dull, drowsy and tired. They may have a fever with chilliness. There is a watery discharge from the nose which irritates and reddens the upper lip and nose. The cough covered by Gels will be croupy, hoarse, barking and have soreness of the chest. The rash will be very itchy and red, in fact, it can be a livid red color. The child may complain of severe pain at the back of the head, heavy eyelids and have a dark red face. There may be chills running up and down the back and you may see them trembling.

◆ Kalium bichromicum (Kali-bi) 30C

The child will likely have a deep loud cough, with expectoration of stringy, yellowish mucus. There may be intense conjunctivitis which can progress to an inflammation of the cornea (keratitis) with ulcers on the surface. The child may complain of pain in the ear which extends into their head and neck. Often there is watery diarrhea with pain on attempting the bowel movement. The throat may be very painful and have ulcers. When the measles is complicated with bronchitis and Bry has not helped, this remedy may be very helpful. It is one of the main remedies to consider if there are ulcers or pus filled vesicles on the cornea of the eye.

✦ Lachesis muta (Lach) 30C

Lach has a very livid rash that is so dark it may look black. There may be a black or dark brown coating on the tongue, lips, teeth and gums, especially if they are dehydrated. The child will often be worse on awakening from sleep, even from a nap. They may be quite talkative even though they are sick.

✦ Mercurius solubilis (Merc) 30C

This is a remedy to think of in measles especially if there are gastrointestinal symptoms present such as diarrhea of foul smelling slimy stools, abdominal pain, indigestion or nausea. The tongue is often heavily coated and imprints of the teeth can be seen along the edge. They may have increased salivation with very bad breath. Bronchitis may be present with a loose barking cough and no expectoration. The child will often be very sweaty and the perspiration will have strong smell. Frequently you will notice swollen glands of throat and difficulty in swallowing.

✦ Pulsatilla pratensis (Puls) 30C

Puls is a remedy often needed in later stages. There may be mucus and congestion. If there is a cough, it will be quite dry at night and looser in the daytime and the child must sit up to cough. The eyes can become crusty along lids and there may be discharge from the eyes. Ear pain is a common symptom. The rash can be slow to come out and when it does it is more dark red than bright red. The spots may have pus. There is dryness of the mouth and lips and the child licks their lips constantly to moisten them but they will not really be thirsty or ask for a drink. There can be a thick yellow discharge from nose. In general, the child will be worse if overheated and may feel better in the cool open air. They can be weepy and clingy, hard to please, and not want to be left alone.

✦ Zincum metallicum (Zinc) 30C

This is a remedy for a weak child with a minimal rash. The child may lie around, not very present, gritting their teeth. The pupils are frequently dilate and they may squint and roll their eyes. They may cry out in their sleep and wake from sleep as if terrified.

Other Therapies

The following therapies can be used to support healing from this condition:

- Burdock (*Arctium lappa*) poultice to soothe the skin.

- Calendula (*Calendula officinalis*) wash to soothe skin and promote healing

- Soaking bath with baking soda, cornstarch or oats to soothe skin.

- Aloe vera gel, chickweed (*Stellaria media*) poultice, lavender (*Lavandula spp.*) poultice or oil topically soothe the skin.

- Clean eyes with warm water or saline if they have conjunctivitis or other eye irritation.

- A humidifier or steam inhalation using any of the previously mentioned essential oils can be supportive to reduce cough and nasal congestion.

1 Centers for Disease Control and Prevention. "Measles (Rubeola) For Healthcare Professionals." cdc.gov. https://www.cdc.gov/measles/hcp/index.html (accessed February 1, 2017).

2 Centers for Disease Control and Prevention. "Epidemiology and Prevention of Vaccine-Preventable Diseases Measles ." cdc.gov. https://www.cdc.gov/vaccines/pubs/pinkbook/meas.html (accessed February 1, 2017).

3 Ibid

4 Centers for Disease Control and Prevention. "Measles (Rubeola) Measles Cases and Outbreaks." cdc.gov. https://www.cdc.gov/measles/cases-outbreaks.html (accessed February 1, 2017).

5 Ibid

6 Ibid

7 Centers for Disease Control and Prevention. "Measles (Rubeola) For Healthcare Professionals." cdc.gov. https://www.cdc.gov/measles/hcp/index.html (accessed February 1, 2017).

8 Price, Shirley, and Len Price. 2015. *Aromatherapy for health professionals.* Edinburgh [etc.]: Churchill Livingstone. 90-91

Chapter 16:
Meningitis

Meningitis is a condition referring to the inflammation of the meninges (a thin tissue covering the spinal cord). It can occur from either a bacterial or viral infection that becomes invasive. Fungal and parasitic infections rarely cause meningitis. Meningococcal disease is caused by a bacteria known as *Neisseria meningitides* (meningococcus). This is an infection of the meninges accompanied by infection of the blood, high fever, stiff neck and headache.[1] Nausea, vomiting, sensitivity to light and mental confusion can be seen as well. Infants less than one year old may not show any of those symptoms but instead may be slow to respond, irritable, inactive, vomiting or poorly feeding.[2] In 2015, there were 375 cases of meningococcal disease of which 10% were fatal.[3]

Infants less than one year of age are at highest risk of infection with meningococcus.[4] One in ten people carry this bacteria in the back of their nose and throat and do not have nor develop any symptoms. Anywhere from 75–85% of children develop natural antibodies to it by adulthood. It is not easily transmitted since it requires long continuous exposure (as in

Meningitis

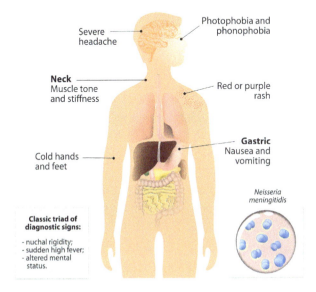

Severe headache

Photophobia and phonophobia

Neck
Muscle tone and stiffness

Red or purple rash

Cold hands and feet

Gastric
Nausea and vomiting

Neisseria meningitidis

Classic triad of diagnostic signs:

- nuchal rigidity;
- sudden high fever;
- altered mental status.

kissing or direct coughing) to infect another person. Airborne droplets alone will not cause infection.[5]

Infants most at risk live in crowded conditions with an affected person. Long term risks and complications include nerve or brain damage, loss of limb, and/ or hearing loss.[6]

Conventional medical doctors will treat children with meningitis immediately with antibiotics. To date, the antibiotics used for it are known to be effective, however, even with antibiotic treatment, 10 to 15 out of every 100 people with meningococcal disease have died from illness complications.

A Vitalistic Naturopathic Approach

> **This is a condition we suggest you not work with at home on your own and we strongly encourage parents to work with their health care provider. The following information is intended to be used by medical professionals. This information is not congruent with the standard care of conventional medicine. Naturopathic doctors, integrative physicians or other holistically trained physicians are the best practitioners to work with using these modalities.**

Basic naturopathic support includes bed rest, broths, oxymel, vitamin A, C and D, zinc, ginger tea, probiotics, garlic or magic socks, medicinal baths, hydrotherapy, dry skin brushing, lymphatic massage, steam inhalation, mushrooms and NAC. If you haven't already reviewed Part 3, that is the section where we discuss these therapies at length. The following suggestions are specific for working with meningitis.

Herbs

+ Antiviral herbs (viral meningitis) such as elderberry (*Sambucus nigra*), astragalus (*Astragalus membranaceus*), echinacea (*Echinacea angustifolia* and/or *Echinacea purpurea*), osha (*Ligusticum porteri*) can be consumed as glycerites.

+ Antibacterial herbs (bacterial meningitis) like goldenseal (*Hydrastis canadensis*), barberry (*Berberis vulgaris*), Oregon grape root (*Mahonia aquifolium*), coptis (*Coptis chinensis*).

Because of their taste, they are best consumed as glycerites

Essential Oils

The primary essential oil known to directly address meningitis is sage (*Salvia officinalis*).[7] It is best used as an inhalation.

Other essential oils known to have broad antiviral properties:

- *Ravensara aromatica*

- Cinnamon (*Cinnamomum verrum*)

- Summer savory (*Saturiea hortensis*)

- Winter savory (Saturiea montana)

- Thyme (*Thymus vulgaris*) ct geraniol and linalool

Ravensara could be used for steam inhalation but the rest are generally too caustic for steam inhalation. For ALL essential oils: avoid using a cold diffuser that runs continuously. Long term (e.g. more than 45–60 minutes), ongoing exposure to any essential oil stresses the liver's detoxification pathways, particularly for young children. Ongoing exposures also increases the risk of sensitizing your child to that essential oil in particular and to essential oils in general.

Topical application:

- One drop each of sage, ravensara, cinnamon and thyme essential oils in one tablespoon of pure, organic vegetable oil. Rub into the soles of the feet and the neck region. You may also add one drop of lavender essential oil to reduce pain, soothe, and promote rest.

- For children under six years old: add one drop of sage, ravensara, cinnamon, thyme and lavender essential oils to three tablespoons of pure, organic vegetable oil.

Homeopathy

Again, as we stated at the beginning, this is a condition we suggest you not work with at home on your own and we strongly encourage parents to work with their health care provider. Homeopathic treatment can be very effective under the care of a doctor properly trained to use this modality.

A child with meningitis will often exhibit a high fever, stiff neck and headache. Other symptoms may include nausea, vomiting, sensitivity to light and mental confusion. Infants less than one year old may not show any of those symptoms but instead may be slow to respond, irritable, inactive, vomiting or poorly feeding. The remedies listed here describe additional unique symptoms your child may have.

The easiest way to choose the remedy you think may work is to compare the list of symptoms you have made for your child to those listed under each remedy. Pick the one that seems to be the best match. For more explanation on how to create a list of symptoms, refer to the homeopathy section in Part 2 of this book.

The following remedies are the most common for this condition but keep in mind that the best remedy for your child may not be listed here. Again, we strongly encourage parents to work with their health care provider.

- **Meningococcinum 30C:**

  Used in the homeopathic prophylactic protocol to help reduce the risk and severity of symptoms.

- **Aconitum napellus (Acon) 30C**

  This remedy is useful at the onset of symptoms. Fear is a marked symptom and is accompanied by restlessness, dry skin, intense thirst and a great fear of death.

- **Apis mellifica (Apis) 30C**

  A remedy often considered for spinal meningitis with inflammation of the serous membranes and disorders with the collection of fluid in tissues and cavities of the body. There may be swellings that look like formations of water-filled sacs. The complaints may be right-sided or midine. There is a general worsening of symptoms from being in a warm room. Being touched also makes the child worse. This remedy covers irritation of the meninges, especially from suppressed eruptions. There are stabbing burning pains like the sting of a bee. The child may put a hand to the head or bore its head into the pillow. The stomach can be sore. The urine may be decreased. The child is often thirstless. There is frequently vomiting of food and a craving for milk. They are better from open air, cold bathing and cold weather. This remedy is useful in every kind of inflammation and swelling worse from exposure to heat or heat application.

Striking symptoms:

- heat in head with throbbing, pressing pains better with pressure and worse on motion

- sudden stabbing pain in head

- dull, heavy sensation in the occiput as if from a blow, extending to neck, better with pressure

- child bores head into pillow due to pain and screams out

- brain feels very tired

- vertigo with sneezing, worse lying down or closing the eyes

- **Belladonna (Bell) 30C**

  Bell is useful in the initial stages with intense heat of body, strong pulse, bright red face and delirium. Cerebral irritation shows up as an intense pain in the head, starting out of sleep with crying out and grinding the teeth. The child is disproportionate sensitive to touch, noises, light and cold air. There is a sudden and rapid rise in temperature.

- **Bryonia alba (Bry) 30C**

  In Bry, there is a high temperature (103+), increased perspiration, white tongue and sharp pains in the head. The child and child's symptoms are worse from any motion and better when lying down and remaining still. There may be an intense bursting headache which is worse when they get up from lying or sitting. There is great thirst with a desire to drink large amounts at one time.

  Striking symptoms:

  - a bursting and splitting headache as if everything would be pressed out as if hit by a hammer from within

  - head pain is worse on motion, stooping, opening the eyes

  - head pain at the back of the head (occiput)

- drawing pain in the bones towards the cheek bones

- head pain along with pain in eyeballs, worse on motion, worse on moving the eyes

- **Camphora officinalis (Camph) 30C**

  There is a sudden onset of symptoms, like a thunderbolt, followed by collapse. The child is cold and pale with a faint pulse and sunken eyes. Even though the child is cold they do not want to be covered.

- **Cuprum aceticum (Cupr-act) 30C**

  In Cup we can see attacks of extreme anguish like fear of death. There is restlessness, groaning and desire to escape or get away although they will not know what they are trying to get away from. There can be vertigo on reading and on looking into the air. They may have a painful sensation as if the head were empty. There is pain in the parietal bone and they will cry out and put their hand on it. There may be a bruised sensation in the brain and the eyes which is worse on moving eyes. There is swelling of the head with redness of the face. They may hold their head at a funny angle either to one side or to one side and backwards. The head may be drawn to one side or falls forward. The symptoms are worse from touch. There may be a purplish-red swelling of the head, face and purple-red or blue lips. Convulsion and twitches in the limbs may be present and are worse when the child is touched.

  Striking symptoms:

  - violent throbbing and lancinating pains in the forehead

  - head seems empty or as if brain were missing

  - vertigo when looking up, especially at a high ceiling

  - heaviness in the head with burning, stinging and stitching pains in the temples and forehead

- **Glonoinum (Glon) 30C**

  The symptoms calling for Glon are frequently pulsating and throbbing in the head, blood vessels and throughout body.

Complaints are worse from the heat of the sun, hot weather, movement and having the hair cut, touched or brushed. The child is better at rest and in the fresh air. The head pain is intense and there is nothing that brings relief. They may "lose their way" in familiar surroundings such as forgetting how to get to the bathroom. There is a heaviness in the forehead and a headache with warm perspiration on forehead. The pulse may be faster than normal and the face red. There is fullness in the head as if the brain were expanding itself. The child may cry out in pain when walking as every step is felt in the neck or when moving the head. The symptoms and pains are better when they are sitting still, lying down and from pressure so they may hold their head in their hands. They may complain of a sore or bruised feeling in the brain which is worse when they shake their head.

◆ Helleborus niger (Hell) 30C

The symptoms of Hell include laziness, headache, screaming or sudden crying out. They may wrinkle the forehead and randomly move one arm and one leg. There are shooting pains in the head which make them cry out suddenly, scream or bore their head into the pillow. The cries have a pitiful sound. The pupils may be dilated and they may sit staring out into space. Typically, the child and their symptoms are from cold air, being uncovered, with exertion and at night, between 4–8 PM. Conversely, they are better in a warm room, being wrapped up and when lying quietly at rest and undisturbed.

Striking symptoms:

- ◆ bores head into the pillow; beats it with hands

- ◆ dull pain in the occiput with sensation of water swashing inside in case of hydrocephalus

- ◆ headache culminates in vomiting

- ◆ rolls head day and night moaning, sudden screams

◆ Veratrum viride (Verat-v) 30C

Often in Verat-v there is an Intense fever with twitching of the body, especially during sleep. There may be an intense cerebral congestion which brings on violent, rapidly appearing headaches with a bursting pain. The heartbeat is slow and weak. There may be coldness of the skin with loss of consciousness and dilated pupils. Vertigo with nausea and sudden weakness may be present. They may vomit after getting up from lying in bed or sitting in the chair. They feel better when they close their eyes and rest their head. The child may complain it is dark since a symptom of this remedy is dim vision. There may be constant jerking or nodding of the head.

- **Zincum metallicum (Zinc) 30C**

  This child may make chewing motions with their mouth and because of sharp pains they bore their head into the pillow. You may see random motions of one arm and one leg. There is a continued state of confusion and cloudiness in the head. Vertigo deep in the brain may cause the child to fall sideways, often to the left. There can be vertigo where the child cannot see and this is worse in the morning, in a warm room and after eating and better in open air. The head pains can be accompanied by nausea and vomiting. The forehead may be cool while the base of the brain at the back of the head is hot. In general the head pains are better in the open air and worse after eating, in a room and in bed.

  Striking symptoms:

  - presence of vertigo and pressing/compressive pains

  - tosses head from side to side

  - bores head into pillow

  - occipital pain with weight on vertex

  - automatic motion of head and hands

  - forehead is cold and base of brain is hot

Other Therapies

  - Constitutional hydrotherapy can support overall immune function and promote healing and recovery.

1 Centers for Disease Control and Prevention. "Meningococcal Disease." cdc. gov. https://www.cdc.gov/meningococcal/index.html (accessed February 1, 2017).

2 Centers for Disease Control and Prevention. "Meningococcal Disease Surveillance." cdc.gov. https://www.cdc.gov/meningococcal/about/symptoms. html (accessed February 1, 2017).

3 Centers for Disease Control and Prevention. "Meningococcal Disease Surveillance." cdc.gov. https://www.cdc.gov/meningococcal/surveillance/ index.html (accessed February 1, 2017).

4 Centers for Disease Control and Prevention. "Meningococcal Disease: Technical and Clinical Information." cdc.gov. https://www.cdc.gov/ meningococcal/clinical-info.html (accessed February 1, 2017).

5 Centers for Disease Control and Prevention. "Meningococcal Disease Causes and Spread to Others." cdc.gov. https://www.cdc.gov/meningococcal/about/ causes-transmission.html (accessed February 1, 2017).

6 Centers for Disease Control and Prevention. "Meningococcal Disease: Technical and Clinical Information." cdc.gov. https://www.cdc.gov/ meningococcal/clinical-info.html (accessed February 1, 2017).

7 Price, Shirley, and Len Price. 2015. *Aromatherapy for health professionals.* Edinburgh [etc.]: Churchill Livingstone. 90-91

Chapter 17:
Mumps

Mumps is a paramyxovirus in the same group as parainfluenzae. It is a contagious virus with a single strand RNA genome. It is transmitted via contact with infected saliva and respiratory secretions. Kissing or sharing utensils, cups, lipstick or cigarettes with an infected person can transmit the virus.[1] Boys are more commonly affected. It is seen more often in camps, colleges and schools.

From January 1st-May 20th, 2017, there were 3,176 cases of mumps in forty-two states and Washington D.C.[2] Historically, cases have ranged from a couple hundred to a couple thousand. For example, in 2012 there were 229 cases; in 2016 there were 5,833 cases. None of the cases that occurred in 2012 were fatal and most happened in college dorms where students were living in crowded conditions.[3]

Mumps is rarely a serious disease. Like measles, a shift has occurred due to vaccinations from early childhood to children over age ten with greater risks for complications associated with an older age group.

Risks and complications of the infection are rare. They are generally seen in adults. Orchitis (inflammation of the testicles occurred in 3–10% of males) but it does not lead to sterility with either one or both testicles affected; less than 1% of cases leads to oophoritis (inflammation of the ovaries); and less than 1% of cases end in deafness, pancreatitis or meningitis. Death from mumps is extremely rare.[4]

Mumps is a viral infection infection of the parotid glands and creates painful swelling in one or both of parotid glands (located beneath ears). Earlobes may be pushed forward from the swelling. There can be pain beneath the ears and swelling in the jaw leading to painful eating and drinking. The incubation period (exposure to appearance of symptoms) is typically 14–28 days. Pain behind the angle of the jaw is usually the first symptom and this may be accompanied by stiffness and soreness on movement. A child will often complain that it hurts to open the mouth and to eat. There may be a slight fever and chills, shivering and sore throat. It often begins on one side and may or may not spread to the other side. The parotid gland can swell quite large but after 4-5 days starts to return to normal size. Other symptoms that may be seen are headache, loss of appetite, muscle aches and fatigue. Keep in mind that about 1/3 of cases have no swelling and or no symptoms. The entire duration of mumps is typically 7–14 days depending on how it is treated.

There are no conventional medical treatments available for mumps.

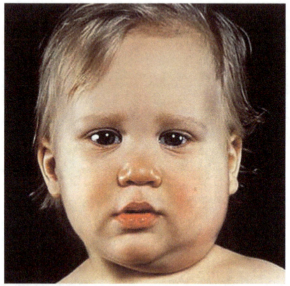

Photo attribution:
http://www.mayoclinic.org/diseases-conditions/mumps/multimedia/mumps/img-20007693

Vitalistic Naturopathic Approach

Basic naturopathic support includes bed rest, broths, oxymel, vitamin A, C and D, zinc, ginger tea, probiotics, garlic or magic socks, medicinal baths, hydrotherapy, dry skin brushing, lymphatic massage, steam inhalation, mushrooms and NAC. If you haven't already reviewed Part 3, that is the section where we discuss these therapies at length. General care tips to keep in mind with measles are: bed rest, a soft diet and localized cold packs. The following suggestions are specific for working with mumps.

Herbs

- Antiviral herbs (viral meningitis) such as elderberry (*Sambucus nigra*), astragalus (Astragalus membranaceus), echinacea (*Echinacea angustifolia* and/or *Echinacea purpurea*), osha (*Ligusticum porteri*) can be consumed as glycerites.

- Cleavers (*Galium aparine*) as a glycerite promotes lymphatic drainage.

- Mullein (*Verbascum thapsus*) as a tea to soothe sore throats.

- Turmeric milk to ease inflammation.

- Slippery elm (*Ulmus fulva*) lozenges to soothe sore throats.

Supplements

- Anti-inflammatory nutrients like bromelain (an enzyme) and fish oils.

- Vitamin A flush: This is a treatment that can be highly effective but should be done under the supervision of a naturopathic physician or other qualified health care practitioner.

Essential Oils

Mumps affects glands in the face and neck area causing painful swelling that in turn blocks lymphatic flow in that region.

- Bay laurel (*Laurus nobilis*) moves lymphatic circulation, which, in turn, can help relieve some of the pain and discomfort associated with mumps.[5]

- Lavender (*Lavandula angustifolia*) can help reduce the pain associated with the swelling and promote relaxation and rest.

- Combine one drop each of bay laurel and lavender in one teaspoon of pure, organic vegetable oil. Rub into the soles of the feet, the jaw and the neck.

- For children under six years old, dilute one drop of bay laurel and one drop of lavender essential oil in two teaspoons of pure, organic vegetable oil. Rub into the soles of the feet, the jaw and the neck.

Homeopathy

A child with mumps will often complain first about pain behind the angle of the jaw, on either or both sides. There may be stiffness and soreness on movement and pain when they open their mouth. There may be a slight fever and chills, shivering and sore throat. The symptoms often start on one side and may or may not spread to the other side. The parotid gland can swell quite large but after 4-5 days starts to return to normal size. Other symptoms that may be seen are headache, loss of appetite, muscle aches and fatigue. Keep in mind that about 1/3 of cases have no swelling and or no symptoms. The remedies listed here describe additional unique symptoms your child may have.

The easiest way to choose the remedy you think may work is to compare the list of symptoms you have made for your child to those listed under each remedy. Pick the one that seems to be the best match. For more explanation on how to create a list of symptoms, refer to the homeopathy section in Part 2 of this book.

The following remedies are the most common for this condition but keep in mind that the best remedy for your child may not be listed here. If you're having difficulty choosing a remedy, consider working with a homeopathic or naturopathic doctor to choose the best remedy.

- **Parotidinum (Parot) 30C:**

  Used in the homeopathic prophylactic protocol to help reduce the risk and severity of symptoms.

- **Aconitum napellus (Acon) 30C**

  This is a remedy most useful at the beginning stages of mumps when there has been a sudden onset of fever, restlessness, anxiety and great thirst. There may be right or left sided swellings of the parotid glands. The child may be fearful.

- **Arsenicum album (Ars) 30C**

  The mumps covered by Ars will usually present with burning pains in the swollen parotid glands or throat that come and go. The child is usually anxious, restless and without their normal energy levels. They will be thirsty and ask for cold water which they will sip at frequent intervals. The pain and inflammation of parotid glands will be better with warm or hot applications.

- **Belladonna (Bell) 30C**

  The swelling of the parotid gland will often be intense, sudden, with redness and violent shooting pains. The child's face is usually flushed with red eyes and a high (103+) fever. This remedy is especially useful when the mumps is accompanied by cerebral symptoms such as delirium, convulsions, unconsciousness or mania coming on after mumps. Often it is the right side which is more affected but it can be both sides.

- **Calcarea carbonica (Calc-c) 30C**

  The child needing Calc-c will often be very sweaty even if there is no fever. Their hands and feet will be cold and damp and their pillow may be damp on first falling asleep. Often the swollen parotids will be firm, almost hard, but if not, that does not mean Calc-c is not the right remedy. The pupils may be dilated and the child may have a sensitivity to light. The swellings can be on either side.

- **Jaborandi (Jab) 30C**

  There is usually a greatly increased amount of saliva which can resemble egg white in consistency. There is increased perspiration which is followed by great thirst after the sweat and salivation have stopped. The child will usually be very drowsy. The face may be red or flushed. The swellings can be on either side.

- **Lachesis muta (Lach) 30C**

  Most frequently this is a left sided swelling or at least the swelling started on the left. The parotid gland is enormously swollen and is very sensitive to touch or pressure. It may be a very dark red or purplish color. The child may have a feeling as if something were swollen in the throat which must be swallowed. However, it is difficult and painful to swallow especially saliva and liquids. The face is red and swollen and the eyes glassy and wild. Pains are aggravated at night and especially on waking up in the morning or after a nap.

- **Mercurius solubilis (Merc) 30C**

  In Merc, the glands are hard, swollen and painful and the pain is worse when blowing the nose. The bones in the face might ache. This is primarily a right side swelling but can be on the left or both sides. There is increased saliva and perspiration similar to Jab but more. Any discharges like breath, sweat, stool, urine and saliva smell bad. The child is worse at night or after lying in bed. They are very sensitive to extremes and changes of temperature. There is an intense thirst in spite of the increased saliva and they may even drool. There may be a bitter or metallic taste in their mouth.

◆ Phytolacca decandra (Phyt) 30C

The throat of a child needed Phyt for mumps will often be very sensitive to the slightest touch. The throat is sore and the pains extend upward toward the ears on swallowing. The throat may also hurt when they stick out their tongue. The parotid and other glands are hard, painful and swollen. There can be increased saliva and sweating, both of which may smell bad. The right side is usually where it starts.

◆ Pilocarpinum +salts (Pilo) 30C

Some homeopaths believe this medicine is the best remedy for the mumps. The main symptoms are excessive salivation and perspiration with a dry mouth. The face is very red. It is more prevalent in the old literature, but it is spoken of highly which is why it has been included although the authors of this book have never found cause to prescribe it.

◆ Pulsatilla pratensis (Puls) 30C

Often, you will be lead to use Puls in this condition because of ear complications following the attack of mumps. The tongue is thickly coated and the mouth is dry but the child is not thirsty. The pain is worse in the evening and after lying down. The children who are sensitive, peevish, chilly and thirstless are especially benefited by this remedy.

◆ Rhus toxicodendron (Rhus-t) 30C

The parotid and submaxillary glands on the right, left or both sides are enormously inflamed and enlarged with this remedy. They can look dark red in color, perhaps are a bit worse on the left side and can feel hard. There may be some pain in the face with a generalized swelling. There may be a cracking motion of the jaw when chewing. The tongue may be coated except the tip (which may be red). Children have great difficulty in opening their mouth. You may see herpes sores on lips. The child is worse from cold air, cold winds and much better from warmth. They like a warm or hot rag on the swollen glands. You will also observe restlessness.

Other Therapies

The following therapies can be used to support healing from this condition.

- Mullein (*Verbascum thapsus*) or Cleavers (*Galium aparine*) poultice to help reduce inflammation and boost local immune function.

- Iodine rub to parotid glands to support local immune function.

- Contrast hydrotherapy to swollen glands to improve local immune function and increase circulation.

1 Centers for Disease Control and Prevention. "Epidemiology and Prevention of Vaccine-Preventable Diseases Mumps." cdc.gov. https://www.cdc.gov/vaccines/pubs/pinkbook/mumps.html (accessed February 1, 2017).

2 Centers for Disease Control and Prevention. "Mumps Cases and Outbreaks." cdc.gov. https://www.cdc.gov/mumps/outbreaks.html (accessed February 1, 2017).

3 Ibid

4 Centers for Disease Control and Prevention. "Mumps for Healthcare Providers." cdc.gov. https://www.cdc.gov/mumps/hcp.html (accessed February 1, 2017).

5 Schnaubelt, Kurt. 1998. *Advanced aromatherapy: the science of essential oil therapy.* Rochester, Vt: Healing Arts Press. 126

Chapter 18:
Pertussis

Pertussis, or whooping cough, is a bacterial contagious disease that most recently peaked in 2012 with just over 48,200 people of all ages infected. The most recent data from 2015 shows 1,833 children less than six months old were infected and 5,876 children between 1-10 years old were infected. It is known to peak every 3–5 years. Interestingly, children with the highest numbers of infection (1,321 children in 2015) had met full compliance of vaccinations (3+ doses) per CDC requirements.[1]

According to the latest CDC statistics, children that had the greatest protection from use of the vaccine had between 1–2 shots.Children that had three shots (the initial shot and two boosters) had the highest rates of pertussis infection (47%). The highest rates of infection reported were for children between the ages of 11–19 years of age. 10% of children known to not have any vaccines acquired whooping cough (269 children between the ages of 1–4 years; sixty children under six months of age). At this point, immunity does not appear to be permanent either through vaccine or infection and antibodies can be present for up to five years.

Because of higher rates of infection in the recent past, the CDC is currently recommending pregnant mothers to obtain the vaccine to confer immunity to fetus. No research on what happens to the fetus when this vaccine is used this way is currently available.

The organism, *Bordetella pertussis*, is spread by being coughed or sneezed on by a person with an active pertussis infection. The bacteria attaches to the cilia (thin, hair-like projections along the respiratory passageways) in the upper respiratory tract and releases a toxin. That toxin causes the airways to swell. It can show up as nosebleeds and eyes hemorrhages from strong coughing fits. It can cause facial swelling, ear infections and decrease oxygen levels in the blood. The worst cases of it can lead to nutritional deficiencies, pneumonia and seizures (causing brain damage).

It is most concerning for children less than six months to a year old because it can be fatal for a child less than one year of age. Even if their life is not threatened, the intense and continual coughing can fatigue a small child. With narrower airways, breathing becomes more difficult and children can go through periods of lack of oxygen. A severe infection can paralyze the respiratory tract.

Pertussis is a contagious infection and so it should be treated as soon as it is suspected. Families that have been able to contain the spread of it have self-quarantined exposed family members until signs and symptoms of the illness have passed.

The incubation period for pertussis is typically 5–10 days. The first symptoms to appear resemble the common cold and include a runny nose, nasal congestion, red, watery eyes, fever, apnea (a pause in breathing) and a mild cough. Unless treated, it can progress to a cough that provokes vomiting, a red or blue face, extreme fatigue and a high-pitched "whoop" sound during intake of air. In milder cases the classic "whooping" cough may not be present. In China, pertussis is known as the "100 day cough" as recovery is often a long process.

The conventional treatment for pertussis infection is to give antibiotics before symptoms appear to prevent the spread of the infection to others. It's important to note that antibiotic treatment does not reduce the severity of the illness. It is not recommended to use antibiotics once infection has set in because larger numbers of bacteria dying release more toxins which worsen paroxysmal coughing. Prescription medicines are used to reduce cough and decrease mucus production.

Videos of Whooping Cough
http://bit.ly/cough1a
http://bit.ly/cough1b
http://bit.ly/cough1c
http://bit.ly/cough1d
http://bit.ly/cough1e

A Vitalistic Naturopathic Approach

Basic naturopathic support includes bed rest, broths, oxymel, vitamin A, C and D, zinc, ginger tea, probiotics, garlic or magic socks, medicinal baths, hydrotherapy, dry skin brushing, lymphatic massage, steam inhalation, mushrooms and NAC. If you haven't already reviewed Part 3, that is the section where we discuss these therapies at length. The following suggestions are specific for working with pertussis.

Herbs

- Berberine containing antibacterial herbs like goldenseal (*Hydrastis canadensis*), barberry (*Berberis vulgaris*), Oregon grape root (*Mahonia aquifolium*), coptis (*Coptis chinensis*). Because of their taste, they are best consumed as glycerites.

- Thyme (*Thymus vulgaris*) is best taken as a tea, glycerite or steam inhalation. It has antimicrobial (antiviral and antibacterial) effects.

- Osha (*Ligusticum porteri*) is best taken as a tea or glycerite. It supports respiratory function and eases spasms.

- Elderberry (*Sambucus nigra*) is best taken as a syrup or glycerite. It is a general immune tonic increasing white blood cell activity and has antibacterial effects.

- Marshmallow root (*Althaea officinalis*) is best taken as a tea or glycerite. It is a safe and effective cough remedy. It contains mucilage and antitussive properties that decrease irritation in the throat due to coughing, reduces inflammation of the lymph nodes, and speeds up recovery from illnesses.

- Lomatium (*Lomatium dissectum*) used as a tea or glycerite is a strong antimicrobial (bacteria and viruses) and has an affinity for the lungs. It stimulates the production of white blood cells, is immunomodulating, enhances production and release of mucus, and eases spasms connected to cough. It is also a nutritive that supports the body during long-standing illness.

- Pleurisy (*Asclepias tuberosa*) as a glycerite to promote expectoration of mucus.

- Elecampane (*Inula helenium*) as a glycerite assists with expectoration, reduces inflammation, is warming to the lungs and is a lung tonic. It has antibacterial, antiviral and antifungal effects.

- Hyssop (*Hyssopus officinalis*) as a glycerite relaxes the smooth bronchial muscles, thins mucus, and eases spasms.

- Yerba Santa (*Eriodictyon californicum/ Eriodictyon angustifolium*) as a tea is used for upper respiratory infections when there is a lot of mucus production. It eases cough, opens up the airways, has antimicrobial (bacteria and viruses) effects, acts as a decongestant, breaks up mucus, and eases coughing spasms.

- Licorice (*Glycyrrhiza glabra*) is an adaptogen (restores normal function) that anti-inflammatory, antioxidant and reduces spasm. It is especially helpful for long-standing illness.

- Herbal Syrup #1: see the Apothecary section for the recipe. It supports the immune system and is antimicrobial.

Supportive Beverages

- Lemon water: It helps clear congestion in the throat, is soothing and is an excellent source of vitamin C.

Essential Oils

Essential oils can be used to soothe the symptoms of whooping cough as well as address the bacteria itself. Choose the oils and the dosage method that are appropriate for your child's age. For ALL essential oils: avoid using a cold diffuser that runs continuously. Long-term (e.g. more than 45–60 minutes), ongoing exposure to any essential oil stresses the liver's detoxification pathways, particularly for young children. Ongoing exposures also increases the risk of sensitizing your child to that essential oil in particular and to essential oils in general.

Newborns to 18 months:

- Breathing in lavender (*Lavandula angustifolia*) essential oil, 1–2 drops on a cotton ball, can soothe the airways in the lungs[2] and also calm the baby.[3] Hold the cotton ball near the baby's nose, avoiding the eyes, for five minutes 2–3 times per day. You also can create an inhaler (see instructions in The Apothecary section at the end of the book).

- Rose (*Rosa damascena*) essential oil has some antimicrobial effects and is very effective in reducing anxiety.[4] Dose by inhaling with a cotton ball or inhaler (see above).

- To help relax and prepare for sleep, combine one drop each of rose and lavender essential oils in two tablespoons of vegetable oil (e.g. organic sunflower oil). Use for full body massage OR rub into the chest and feet only. You can repeat the foot and chest massage if the baby wakes coughing in the night.

18 months- 4 years: all of the above treatments plus:

- Eucalyptus (*Eucalyptus radiata*): 1–2 drops on a cotton ball OR use inhaler. Inhale for at least 5–7 minutes three times a day. Eucalyptus relaxes the bronchi and is effective against a broad range of bacteria,[5] including several antibiotic-resistant bacteria.[6]

* Tea tree (*Melaleuca officinalis*) is effective against a broad range of bacteria as well as viruses and fungi. Tea tree also reduces inflammation.[7] Inhaling tea tree essential oil can help reduce bronchial swelling and spasms. Add 1–2 drops to a cotton ball OR use an inhaler. Inhale for 5–7 minutes three times a day.

* Eucalyptus and tea tree essential oil steam inhalation.

* Tangerine (*Citrus tangerina*) and mandarin (Citrus reticulata) essential oils.

both have antibacterial properties. They also are excellent for brightening moods and reducing anxiety. Add 1–2 drops to a cotton ball and inhale for 5–7 minutes at least three times per day.

5–12+ year olds:

* Spearmint (*Mentha spicata*) has many of the same antibacterial pain relieving characteristics of peppermint (*Mentha piperita*), but is milder and therefore more appropriate for children. Add 1–2 drops to a cotton ball and inhale 5–7 minutes at least three times a day OR use an inhaler.

* Spearmint essential oil steam inhalation to open up respiratory passageways.

* Chest rub with one tablespoon of sunflower or almond oil and one drop each of spearmint, eucalyptus, lavender, chamomile and tea tree essential oils. Rub into the chest throughout the day to soothe lungs and keep airways clear.

* Eucalyptus, spearmint and lavender chest rub. Massage into the chest 3–4 times per day.

Homeopathy

A child with pertussis will likely have a runny nose, nasal congestion, red, watery eyes, fever and apnea (a pause in breathing). The cough can range from mild (early on) to a cough that provokes vomiting, a red or blue face, extreme fatigue and a high-pitched "whoop" sound during intake of air. In addition to these, you will notice that there are more specific qualities that may be unique to what your child is experiencing, especially in regards to what makes their cough better or worse. The remedies listed here describe unique symptoms your child may have.

The easiest way to choose the remedy you think may work is to compare the list of symptoms you have made for your child to those listed under each remedy. Pick the one that seems to be the best match. For more explanation on how to create a list of symptoms, refer to the homeopathy section in Part 2 of this book.

There is no other treatment that can bring about such a dramatic improvement in pertussis as homeopathy. What follows is a list of remedies known to help resolve the condition faster and relieve the troublesome cough. This is not a list of all known remedies, only the most common.

Keep in mind that the best remedy for your child may not be listed here. If you're having difficulty choosing a remedy, consider working with a homeopathic or naturopathic doctor to choose the best remedy.

- **Pertussinum (Pert) 30C:**

    Used in the homeopathic prophylactic protocol to help reduce the risk and severity of symptoms.

- **Aconitum napellus (Acon) 30C**

    A remedy useful when the illness has come on suddenly and associated symptoms are fever, chilliness, and restlessness or fear. The face may be red or pale in color and the pulse is often rapid. There is a short, dry, intense cough with a loud and sharp quality. The cough is typically worse at night and worse around midnight. These children can feel better and the cough is better in the open air, but symptoms will have begun after exposure to dry, cold air. There may be a level of fear and anxiety present that is much greater than what you would expect.

- **Antimonium tartaricum (Ant-t) 30C**

    If a cough is present it often sounds rattly but hardly any mucus comes up. It sounds like there is a lot to cough up, so much that it seems almost like the child will drown in his/ her own fluids. The cough is often worse from 10 PM until midnight, worse after eating and lying down. The cough will be in paroxysms and the child is often breathless and exhausted afterwards. The coughing effort to bring up the mucus may result in vomiting. The child is usually cross, irritable, and weak from efforts to raise the phlegm. There may be incredible mood changes that swing from relatively pleasant to very unpleasant, almost like Dr. Jekyll and Mr. Hyde.

◆ Arnica (Arn) 30C

Arn is helpful to relieve the pain from the coughing fits which can be violent and lead to a bruised sensation in the ribs.

◆ Belladonna (Bell) 30C

This remedy is often called for in the early feverish stages of pertussis. If it is the correct remedy and used early enough, it can change the course of the illness. The coughing stage comes on suddenly and is often violent. The child can have a red face, bulging eyes, dilated pupils and abdominal pain. Between the coughing fits, there is often a pronounced tickling in the larynx until the next bout of coughing. There can be a severe headache with throbbing pains with the cough. There may be a very sore, red and swollen throat, and loss of the voice.

◆ Bromium (Brom) 30C

The child may have a croupy cough that is very spasmodic and have hard glands in the neck. They have a sore throat and may lose their voice or sound very hoarse. The cough is worse in warm damp air (in the shower). The child and cough may be better with exercise or movement and with occupation (when playing or busy).

◆ Bryonia alba (Bry) 30C

The child will have a dry cough which hurts the head and chest. Because the head hurts, the child will hold the head or chest with his or her hands when coughing. This is a very severe cough and there may be complaints of pressure over the sternum and painful breathing. When the child coughs it seems as if the entire body shakes. The child wants to lie perfectly still as the slightest motion causes intense pain on breathing. The child prefers to lie on the painful side, but this is related to movement making the pains worse. The cough is worse when entering a warm room from the outside cold air. If it is not cold outside, then it may be worse on entering a room warmer than the one the child was in. The lips are dry and the tongue is dry and coated. The child is thirsty for large quantities of water at long intervals. Any mucus that is coughed up has a bitter taste.

◆ Coccus cacti (Cocc-c) 30C

If the child is producing mucus it will be clear, thick and ropey. There is a choking cough that can result in vomiting of long strings of mucus that hang from the mouth and nose. In fact, they may complain that there is something in their throat, cough and keep coughing until they gag and vomit. Drinking cold water may bring temporary relief from tickling in the larynx and the coughing spells. The spells may become worse early in the morning and/or around 11–11:30 p.m. This thick ropey mucus is more white than the thick ropey mucus of Kali-bi which would be more yellow.

◆ Corallium rubrum (Cor-r) 30C

The child may feel a smothering sensation before the cough. This can look like a gasping and crowing as they try to take a breathe and they may become dark blue / black in the face. This is a remedy particularly for a cough that is short, quick and ringing, often called a "minute gun" cough. After the coughing spell, the child is exhausted. No other remedy covers such a violent coughing spell as well. It is said to be indicated in the later stages of pertussis.

◆ Cuprum (Cupr) 30C

The coughing fits covered by this remedy are rapid, last a long time and are very distressful for the child. If the coughing episodes result in gasping for air or difficulty breathing and end in exhaustion, Cup is highly indicated. You may see cramps, muscular spasms, clenched fists, and/or convulsions with the cough. Violent coughing may lead to a blue discoloration of the face and around the lips. Cold drinks of water may bring dramatic but temporary relief from the coughing attacks. The cough may wake the child around 3 a.m.

where he or she sits up suddenly gasping for air.

◆ Drosera (Dros) 30C

The coughing fits of Drosera are extreme and can cause a blue face and lips. The fit can be so extreme that the child may act or feel as if suffocating. The cough is violent and the child may have gagging, retching or vomiting following the coughing fits. The child will prefer and be better with cold drinks. Cramps in the hands and feet during coughing may be present. The cough will often be worse at night.

◆ Hepar sulphuris calcarea (Hep) 30C

This may be a child who has a tendency for recurrent croup. The cough is typically dry and worse in the evening. There can be sharp pains in the throat or chest and the pain can make the child irritable. In general, this child may be oversensitive to pain and complains intensely. The child often does not want to be touched by anyone and if they are touched the symptoms are worse. The child and child's symptoms are also worse from cold air or drafts of air. The skin can be extremely sensitive to moving air. The cough may improve from being in a hot steamy bathroom or after a shower. This symptom is not always present but is important when present.

◆ Iodium (Iod) 30C

This is another excellent remedy for pertussis. The child is usually very hot and has a lot of energy but the symptoms tend to worsen when they become overheated. The cough is dry, intense and spasmodic. There may be a high and prolonged fever. The larynx will feel tight and constricted. The child may not be able to say any more than the neck feels tight or squeezed. Children who would benefit from this remedy usually have strong energy, and now appear very weak and wrung out with illness. Like Brom, the neck glands tend to be swollen and hard.

◆ Kali bichromicum (Kali-bi) 30C

The cough of Kali-bi is very hoarse. The child's breathing may be superficial and rapid in an attempt to prevent cough. There may be stringy yellow-green mucus that is difficult to expel from the throat. The child will repeatedly cough and finally bring up a small amount of mucus, again, often stringy. They may also have thick stringy mucus in the nose.

♦ Magnesia Phosphorica (Mag-p) 30C

The condition often begins as what looks like the common cold. In the early stages there may only be a few symptoms but once the cough sets in the attacks are convulsive and nervous and end in a classical whoop sound. The face may also turn blue or swollen and red.

♦ Phosphorus (Phos) 30C

Phos is a very common remedy in pertussis. There may be recurrent nosebleeds with the coughing, increased thirst, fever, sore throat and general weakness. There may be a sense of heaviness or tightness in the chest, a dry cough, hoarseness or loss of voice. The child may complain of hot or burning pains when coughing or when describing the pain in the throat. Breathing is difficult and the child says they cannot get enough air. The chest wall may heave, nostrils may flare and the child is obviously having difficulty breathing. The child may be shaky with twitching facial muscles. There is a tormenting, irritating cough accompanied by rawness or burning in the chest. They will want cold or sweet things to eat but may experience nausea shortly after eating or drinking. The child needing this remedy will be much better when consoled or held by the parent. This child does not want to be left alone and may become very distressed when a parent leaves the room. The child may be very fearful or anxious that something bad is going to happen in general or to a loved one.

♦ Pulsatilla pratensis (Puls) 30C

The cough of Puls is dry, teasing (constant tickle) and worse in the evening and at night. The child must sit up in bed to get relief. There is a loose cough in the morning, with much mucus and expectoration. The cough is worse in a warm room or when entering a warm room. The child is worse when heated and in a closed up room and will want the windows and doors open. The expectoration is thick, bland, yellowish-green and bitter. The child may complain of soreness, pressure or tightness on the chest. Urine may spurt when coughing. The child needing Puls when sick is often tearful, timid and likes sympathy. There is usually a decreased level of hunger and almost no thirst.

- **Rumex (Rum) 30C**

  The cough covered by Rum is dry, constant, violent and fatiguing. There is a tickling in the notch at the top of the sternum. The cough is worse in the evening, at night, after lying on left side and upon touching or pressing the pit of the throat. The cough is often triggered from breathing cold air and can be worse when going from a warm to a cold room. The child may want to cover the nose and mouth when breathing. A few drops of urine may be passed when coughing. One way to tell if this remedy is a good choice is to open the freezer door and have the child take a deep breath. If it triggers the cough, this may be a good place to start.

- **Spongia tosta (Spong) 30C**

  Spong may be one of the most widely used remedies for croup. The cough can be dry and barky or it can sound hollow, almost like a saw going through wood. In general, dryness is a theme. Dry mouth, dry membranes, dry tongue and dry eyes dominate the symptoms. There can also be a burning sensation along with the sensation of dryness. The cough is especially worse just before midnight. The child will complain of a tickle or crumb sensation in the area of the voice box which is worse when they inhale. The cough is often worse and a coughing fit can be triggered when inhaling. The cough is worse if the child overheats but is usually improved with a warm drink or after eating. It is worse with a cold drink. The child may have increased anxiety or act uncharacteristically fearful.

Other therapies

The following therapies can be used to support healing from this condition.

- Herbal Steam inhalations: herbs such as lavender, eucalyptus, calendula or thyme can be used to support respiratory function and reduce infection

- Saltwater and colloidal silver gargle: two years or older (must be able to gargle) to help reduce inflammation.

+ Iodine rub to support local immune function.

+ Chest Packs using mustard or onion (see recipes in The Apothecary) to support local immune function, aid respiration and increase circulation.

+ Chest percussion[8]

1 "Notice to Readers: Final 2015 Reports of Nationally Notifiable Infectious Diseases and Conditions". 2016. MMWR. *Morbidity and Mortality Weekly Report.* 65 (46): 1306-1321.

2 Ueno-Iio, Tomoe, Misako Shibakura, Kanayo Yokota, Michinori Aoe, Tomoko Hyoda, Ryoko Shinohata, Arihiko Kanehiro, Mitsune Tanimoto, and Mikio Kataoka. 2014. "Lavender essential oil inhalation suppresses allergic airway inflammation and mucous cell hyperplasia in a murine model of asthma". *Life Sciences.* 108 (2): 109-115.

3 de Sousa DP, de Almeida Soares Hocayen P, LN Andrade, and R Andreatini. 2015. "A Systematic Review of the Anxiolytic-Like Effects of Essential Oils in Animal Models". *Molecules* (Basel, Switzerland). 20 (10): 18620-60.

4 Mahboubi, Mohaddese. 2016. "Rosa damascena as holy ancient herb with novel applications". *Journal of Traditional and Complementary Medicine.* 6 (1): 10-16.

5 Salem, M.Z.M., N.A. Ashmawy, H.O. Elansary, and A.A. El-Settawy. 2015. "Chemotyping of diverse Eucalyptus species grown in Egypt and antioxidant and antibacterial activities of its respective essential oils". *NATURAL PRODUCT RESEARCH.* 29 (7): 681-685.

6 Mulyaningsih S, F Sporer, J Reichling, and M Wink. 2011. "Antibacterial activity of essential oils from Eucalyptus and of selected components against multidrug-resistant bacterial pathogens". *Pharmaceutical Biology.* 49 (9): 893-9.

7 Golab M, and K Skwarlo-Sonta. 2007. "Mechanisms involved in the anti-inflammatory action of inhaled tea tree oil in mice". *Experimental Biology and Medicine* (Maywood, N.J.). 232 (3): 420-6.

8 Medline Plus. "Postural drainage." medlineplus.gov. https://medlineplus.gov/ency/patientinstructions/000051.htm (accessed February 1, 2017).

Chapter 19:
Pneumonia (Pneumococcal)

Pneumonia is a mild to serious condition where cough, fever, shortness of breath, chest pain, nausea, vomiting and weakness can occur. In more severe cases, it can cause fluid to accumulate around the lungs and cause difficulty breathing. Although pneumonia can be caused by bacteria, viruses or fungi, the most common bacteria found in children is *Streptococcus pneumoniae*.[1] It is spread by coming into contact with respiratory droplets from someone carrying the microorganism.

The most recent Active Bacterial Core (ABC) Surveillance figures available from the CDC show that in 2015 there were two cases per 100,000 people with pneumonia due to *S. pneumoniae*.[2, 3] That same year, there were 77 cases of children that were less than one year old, fifty-four one year old children and sixty-five 2-4 year old children affected. There are more than ninety strains of the bacteria that exist and 30% of them are antibiotic resistance (severe cases of pneumonia are due to the antibiotic resistant strains).[4]

Most cases of pneumonia, whether bacterial or viral, begin as what looks like the common cold or flu: sneezing, runny nose, general not-well feeling, muscle aches and pains. Pneumonia can be suspected if there are symptoms such as a fever up to 105° degrees, coughing up green/yellow/bloody phlegm, severe chills, extreme fatigue, perspiration, difficulty breathing, blue lips or fingernails, chest heaviness or pain and rapid heartbeat.

The age group that is most susceptible to infection with *S. pneumoniae* are children that are over three weeks but less than three months old. Children less than two years old are more susceptible to having pneumonia related to viral infections.[5] A note about *S. pneumoniae* is that it is a common inhabitant of the respiratory tract and most children are colonized by the time they are one year of age. If it becomes invasive, it can lead to complications like mild sinus and ear infections (some parents will consider inserting tubes in their children's ears when ear infections are chronic), bacteremia or meningitis. A child with a severe case of meningitis from exposure to *S. pneumoniae* infection can end up with hearing loss or brain damage with developmental delays.

Risk factors that put children at greater risk of infection is exposure to secondhand smoke, not breastfeeding, being in daycare, a recent flu, having a vitamin A deficiency, recent use of antibiotics and being of either African American, Alaskan American or Native American descent.[6,7]

If a child has a bacterial case of pneumonia, antibiotics are the conventional course of treatment. In the case of a severe infection, IV antibiotics may be prescribed. Bacterial pneumonia must be treated as it can lead to serious illness such as sepsis. This is a condition in which parents are strongly encouraged to work with their doctor. Viral pneumonia will clear up on its own if left untreated, although, it can take a long time.

The conventional medical approach is to treat a child with a bacterial case of pneumonia with antibiotics. In the case of *S. pneumoniae,* it has become highly antibiotic resistant and doctors are using a variety of antibiotics to manage it.[8]

For viral cases of pneumonia, conventional medicine doesn't suggest any form of treatment other than keeping a child hydrated. They also advise against using cough suppressants since being able to clear the airways is important.

Vitalistic Naturopathic Approach

Basic naturopathic support includes bed rest, broths, oxymel, vitamin A, C and D, zinc, ginger tea, probiotics, garlic or magic socks, medicinal baths, hydrotherapy, dry skin brushing, lymphatic massage, steam inhalation, mushrooms and NAC. If you haven't already reviewed Part 3, that is the section where we discuss these therapies at length.

Protective factors include breastfeeding and avoiding daycare settings.[9] The wholistic therapies listed below can be used for both viral and bacterial pneumonia and can support the body and speed up the recovery time. When treating bacterial pneumonia, one or more of the antibacterial herbs should be included in the treatment plan.

Herbs

- Lomatium (*Lomatium dissectum*) used as a tea or glycerite is a strong antimicrobial (bacteria and viruses) herb and has an affinity for the lungs. It stimulates the production of white blood cells, is immunomodulating, enhances production and release of mucus and eases spasms connected to cough. It is also a nutritive herb that supports the body during long-standing illness.

- Mullein (*Verbascum thapsus*) as a tea or glycerite soothes the lungs.

- Osha (*Ligusticum porteri*) as a glycerite supports respiratory function.

- Berberine containing antibacterial herbs can be goldenseal (*Hydrastis canadensis*), barberry (*Berberis vulgaris*), oregon grape root (*Mahonia aquifolium*), coptis (*Coptis chinensis*). Because of their taste, they are best consumed as glycerites. Choose one of these herbs.

- Antiviral herbs (viral meningitis) such as elderberry (*Sambucus nigra*), astragalus (*Astragalus membranaceus*), echinacea (*Echinacea angustifolia* and/or *Echinacea purpurea*), osha (*Ligusticum porteri*) can be consumed as glycerites.

- Pleurisy (*Asclepias tuberosa*) as a glycerite to promote expectoration of mucus.

- Elecampane (*Inula helenium*) as a glycerite assists with expectoration, reduces inflammation, is warming to the lungs and is a lung tonic. It has antibacterial, antiviral and antifungal effects.

- Hyssop (*Hyssopus officinalis*) as a glycerite relaxes the smooth bronchial muscles, thins mucus, and eases spasms.

- Yerba Santa (*Eriodictyon californicum/ Eriodictyon angustifolium*) as a tea is used for upper respiratory infections when there is a lot of mucus production. It eases cough, opens up the airways, has antimicrobial (bacteria and viruses) effects, acts as a decongestant, breaks up mucus, and eases coughing spasms.

- Licorice (*Glycyrrhiza glabra*) is an adaptogen (restores normal function) that anti-inflammatory, antioxidant and reduces spasm. It is especially helpful for long-standing illness.

Supplements

- Mushroom formula containing a blend of chaga (*Inonotus obliquus*), cordyceps (*Ophiocordyceps sinensis*), reishi (*Ganoderma lucidum*) and shiitake (*Lentinula edodes*): used as a glycerite or in apple or pear sauce. Mushrooms strengthen and support immune function.

- For viral pneumonia, implement a Vitamin A flush. This is a treatment that can be highly effective but should be done under the supervision of a naturopathic physician or other qualified health care practitioner.

Essential Oils

Essential oils are powerful allies in addressing pneumonia, both by themselves and in combination with antibiotics. As more bacteria are developing resistance to antibiotics, research is demonstrating essential oils can help improve the effectiveness of antibiotics by circumventing the cells' resistance mechanisms.[10] In addition, essential oils have potent antibacterial action in and of themselves.

Recent research demonstrates three essential oils have strong antibacterial action for pneumonia:

- Russian Wormwood (*Artemisia verstita*) for *Klebsiella pneumoniae* infection. In this study, the whole essential oil was more effective than isolated constituents.[11]

- Spotted bee balm (*Monarda punctata*) for *Streptococcus pneumoniae* infection.[12]

- Cinnamon (Cinnamomum zeylanicum) for both *Klebsiella* and *Streptococcus pneumoniae* infections.[13] Be cautious with young children as cinnamon can be very caustic. Use extremely diluted preparations for young children.

Additional essential oils for Klebsiella pneumoniae:

- Helichrysum (*Helichrysum angustifolium*) For Diplococcus pneumoniae, all of the following have strong antibacterial activity:[14]

- Cajeput (*Melaleuca leucadendron*)

- Summer savory (*Satureia hortensis*)

- Winter savory (*Satureia montana*)

- Clove bud (*Syzgium aromaticum*)

For bacterial pneumoniae, the following essential oils have strong antibacterial activity:[15]

◆ Spanish oregano (*Thymus capitatus*)

◆ Thyme (*Thymus vulgaris*)

Additional essential oils that can help address pneumonia:

◆ *Eucalyptus radiata* helps to open the bronchi, expectorate mucus, and reduce inflammation.

◆ Rosemary (*Rosmarinus officinalis*) ct verbenone has mucolytic action.

◆ Bay laurel (Laurus nobilis) helps to expectorate mucus.

External ways to use the essential oils for pneumonia:

◆ Chest and foot rub: choose two or three of the essential oils listed above, as appropriate, for the type of pneumonia present. Repeat application 3–4 times a day. Rotate the combination of essential oils you are using every 2–3 days, to avoid the skin becoming sensitized to the essential oils. Repeat application 3–4 times a day.

◆ Inhaler: Choose one or a combination of the above essential oils.

◆ Steam inhalation: 2–3 drops of *Eucalyptus radiata* essential oil and one drop of summer savory OR other antimicrobial essential oil (see above).

◆ For ALL essential oils: avoid using a cold diffuser that runs continuously. Long-term (e.g. more than 45–60 minutes), ongoing exposure to any essential oil stresses the liver's detoxification pathways, particularly for young children. Ongoing exposures also increases the risk of sensitizing your child to that essential oil in particular and to essential oils in general.

Homeopathy

A child diagnosed with pneumonia will likely have a cough, fever, shortness of breath, chest pain, nausea, vomiting and weakness. The remedies listed here describe additional unique symptoms your child may have.

The easiest way to choose the remedy you think may work is to compare the list of symptoms you have made for your child to those listed under each remedy. Pick the one that seems to be the best match. For more explanation on how to create a list of symptoms, refer to the homeopathy section in Part 2 of this book.

This is broken into sections depending on the stage of the pneumonia. We highly recommend you read the accompanying write up from Dr. Borland which provides the in depth guidance for successful treatment of   pneumonia   https://www.vitalhealthpublishing.com/borland-pneumonia. We also strongly encourage parents and caregivers to work with a professional as pneumonia can become complicated quickly.

Preventative

+ **Pneumococcinum (Pneu) 30C.**

    Used in the homeopathic prophylactic protocol to help reduce the risk and severity of symptoms.

Incipient stage (first 24 hours)

+ **Aconitum napellus (Acon) 30C**

    Typically, a very sudden onset especially after exposure to cold occurs. There is a high temperature, marked excitement, restlessness and acute anxiety. There will be a full, bounding pulse, flushed face, contracted pupils and hot, dry skin. The child may report coldness of the extremities. The mouth may be dry and feels hot and tingling while accompanied by intense thirst for cold drinks. There is a constant, dry, short cough, which the child will say is happening because their throat is dry. The child may have stabbing pains, usually in the left side of the chest. The symptoms are usually worse beginning in the late evening until midnight, thereafter some improvement may be seen.

+ **Belladonna (Bell) 30C**

    There is usually a fast sudden onset like Acon. The attack is always very severe with a violent temperature, up to 105 degrees or higher. The pulse feels as if it would burst through the vessels and the child is extremely excited. The face is bright red with a generalized blush over the whole skin. The skin is often burning hot to touch. The pupils may be dilated and the child may be sensitive to light. The mouth is dry and, although usually thirsty, there may be no thirst. Even if the child is not thirsty, there will be complaints of the mouth being very dry, hot and burning. The tongue is often swollen, dry and dark red. Bell usually covers a right sided pneumonia but can also be on the left or both sides. The cough is a very dry, painful, tearing cough, and the sputum is usually very scanty. The child will have a throbbing headache which is worse if lying with the head flat and better if slightly propped up. The chest wall may become very sensitive to touch and hurts when coughing.

- **Ferrum phosphoricum (Ferr-p) 30C**

  Pneumonia takes longer to develop in children who need Ferr-p than in those who need Acon. Another distinguishing feature between Ferr-p and Acon is instead of the very brightly flushed face and hot, dry skin of Acon, you find either a localized flush over the cheekbones or a variable state of redness (child coughs, is disturbed, or has to talk, then rapidly flushes bright red but resting the flush tends to return to a flush on the cheekbones). There can be paleness around the mouth. The child is tired, does not want to talk, is sensitive to noise and wants to be left alone. Both Acon and Ferr-p run a high temperature, have a rapid, bounding pulse, are very thirsty for cold water. However, the tongue can be different in Acon and Ferr-p. In Acon it is usually dry, and not coated whereas in Ferr-p it can be somewhat swollen. There is a constant tormenting cough in Ferr-p but, instead of being from a sensation of dryness in the throat as in Acon, it is from a sense of irritation lower down behind the sternum. The cough can be accompanied by nosebleeds. The child is sensitive to cold and the cough is worse by a draft of cold air. This pneumonia is more right-sided than left. The child is worse in the early morning 4–6 AM.

- **Ipecacuanha (Ipecac) 30C**

  The ailment almost always starts with vomiting. The onset is slower than with Acon, Ferr-p and Bell. The child usually tends to have a dusky flush, and a hot, sweaty face. The temperature is not so high as in the others, about 103 degrees, and the pulse is less bounding. There is mucus in the chest producing a generalized rattle with spells of coughing that leave the child feeling as if they would suffocate. The coughing can lead to retching with stringy, difficult, bright red bloodstained spit. They are exhausted after the coughing spell. The lips are often pale, almost whitish. The child feels rotten, very sick, does not want to be fussed over. Although the child may ask for something, it is not really want it and will be refused once handed over to the child. There is often nasal irritation with violent attacks of sneezing. The mouth is sticky and the tongue can be either clean or heavily coated. The child is sensitive to a stuffy room, which can bring on the cough, and will desire moving air like a fan blowing directly on the body.

Developed Pneumonia (after first 24 hours)

◆ **Bryonia alba (Bry) 30C**

There is a gradual onset of the pneumonia. The child has been out of sorts for a day or two, then wakes one morning feeling ill. There may have been some sneezing and a stuffed up feeling in the head. This often starts with a shiver and within a few hours a fever develops. The child is congested, heavy and sleepy looking. The face is dusky and the child feels hot and has a hot, damp sweat (not profuse perspiration). Within a day, the extremities may become dusky and the lips turn dusky, dry, cracked and somewhat swollen. There can be an intense frontal headache which settles over the eyes. There is more of a feeling of weight than pain which becomes painful with any movement. The child generally feels extremely ill on sitting up and may even feel faint. There is a heavy thick, white coating on a dry tongue and the mouth feels dry. They are very thirsty for large quantities of cold water. There may be a bitter taste in the mouth. This child dislikes being disturbed at all, resents having to do anything, having to talk and is very short tempered. The child is difficult to satisfy. It is more likely the right lung that is affected but left sided pneumonia can be present as well. Coughs brings intense pain and you may see the child sitting up in bed holding the chest when coughing. Breathing happens by taking short panting breaths, keeping the breath as shallow as possible because any movement of the chest wall hurts. The voice may be hoarse. The child feels hot and is worse in a hot room. The child may be worse at 9 PM.

◆ **Chelidonium majus (Chel) 30C**

The pneumonias in which Bry is used without success may be cases in which Chel should have been used. There is often a dusky appearance with slight yellowish tinge (vs bluish tinge of Bry). This may be a deep flush in the cheeks which may be one-sided (R more common).The child is lethargic and does not want to be disturbed or make any effort to move. They are aggravated by movement and irritable. The irritability is similar to Bry but can be meaner or spiteful in nature. Often, you will see right sided complaints that extend through the body to the back. The tongue is yellowish vs the whitish tongue of Bry. There is much sputum production and expectoration, more than in Bry, and it is easier to bring up in Chel as compared to Bry. There is an intense thirst for hot things in Chel as compared to Bry in which the child prefers cold drinks. The child is better when they sit up and lean forward as compared to Bry in which lying on affected side helps the child feel better. The child is usually worse at either or both 4 AM and 4 PM as compared to Bry where the child is worse around 9 PM.

◆ **Phosphorus (Phos) 30C**

This pneumonia develops more quickly than in Bry. There is a sense of heaviness or tightness in the chest, a dry cough, hoarse voice or loss of voice. The child has a brighter red flush than in Bry which fades when at rest. The skin surface is hot and moist. The child is more awake, worried and anxious than Bry. Breathing is difficult and the child says they cannot get enough air. The chest wall may heave, nose may flare and there is obvious difficulty breathing. Hands may be shaky with twitching of the facial muscles. There is a tormenting irritating cough accompanied by a sensation of rawness or burning in the chest. The tongue tends to be dry, red and a little swollen but can become coated with a light, dry, white or whitish-yellow coating. They will be intensely thirsty for cold drinks and may ask for something juicy or sour rather than plain cold water. They will want to be propped up and you may see them lift their chin or throw their head back to help with breathing. They are often chilly and and a draft of cold air excites the cough. They feel anxiety and fear. They dislike being left alone, are scared if left alone and are much better if someone is nearby holding and comforting them. It is the physical contact that gives relief. The temperature is about 103 degrees with a full, strong pulse.

- **Veratrum viride (Verat-v) 30C**

    In Vert-v there is often a rapid rise of temperature with a high fever (up to 105 degrees). The child has a livid red face with a feeling of intense pulsation, as if the heart were pounding out through the chest wall. When you feel the child's pulse it is full and bounding. There is excitement, in general, and a violent delirium may develop quite early. The child sees faces and figures on the wall. The pupils are widely dilated. There is a lot of perspiration that may appear as beads of sweat (as opposed to Bell, which has dry burning hot skin). The child is very thirsty and often has slight nausea. The child may say that the water tastes "sweet." When you look at the tongue you may see either a thick, yellowish coating or a thick coating with a bright red streak down the center. It is difficult to get the mucus up as it is a little sticky, and there is always a certain amount of chest pain while coughing. The pain is less than the stabbing pain of Bryonia or the raw burning pain of Phosphorus.

Other Therapies

- Iodine or castor oil chest rub to support local immune function and increase circulation.

1 Ostapchuk, M., D. M. Roberts, and R. Haddy. 2004. "Community-Acquired Pneumonia in Infants and Children". *AMERICAN FAMILY PHYSICIAN*. 70 (5): 899-908.

2 Centers for Disease Control and Prevention. "Pneumococcal Disease Surveillance and Reporting." cdc.gov. https://www.cdc.gov/pneumococcal/ surveillance.html (accessed February 1, 2017).

3 Centers for Disease Control and Prevention. "ABCs Report: Streptococcus pneumoniae, 2015." cdc.gov. https://www.cdc.gov/abcs/reports-findings/ survreports/spneu15.html (accessed February 1, 2017).

4 Centers for Disease Control and Prevention. "Pneumococcal Disease Drug Resistance." cdc.gov. https://www.cdc.gov/pneumococcal/drug-resistance. html (accessed February 1, 2017).

5 Ostapchuk, M., D. M. Roberts, and R. Haddy. 2004. "Community-Acquired Pneumonia in Infants and Children". *AMERICAN FAMILY PHYSICIAN*. 70 (5): 899-908.

6 Andrews, H. and H. Zwickey. "The Vaccine Balancing Act" Seminar. 2009.

7 Centers for Disease Control and Prevention. "Epidemiology and Prevention of Vaccine-Preventable Diseases Pneumococcal Disease." cdc.gov. https:// www.cdc.gov/vaccines/pubs/pinkbook/pneumo.html#secular (accessed February 1, 2017).

8 Centers for Disease Control and Prevention. "Pneumococcal Disease Diagnosis and Medical Management." cdc.gov. https://www.cdc.gov/ pneumococcal/clinicians/diagnosis-medical-mgmt.html (accessed February 1, 2017).

9 Pelton, S. I., O. S. Levine, C. A. Van Beneden, and B. Schwartz. 2000. "Risk Factors for Invasive Pneumococcal Disease in Children: A Population-Based Case-Control Study in North America". *PEDIATRICS -SPRINGFIELD-*. 105: 1172.

10 Langeveld WT, EJ Veldhuizen, and SA Burt. 2014. "Synergy between essential oil components and antibiotics: a review". *Critical Reviews in Microbiology*. 40 (1): 76-94.

11 Yang C, DH Hu, and Y Feng. 2015. "Essential oil of Artemisia vestita exhibits potent in vitro and in vivo antibacterial activity: Investigation of the effect of oil on biofilm formation, leakage of potassium ions and survival curve measurement". *Molecular Medicine Reports*. 12 (4): 5762-70.

12 Li, Hong, Yang, Tian, Li, Fei-Yan, Yao, Yan, and Sun, Zhong-Min. 2014. *Antibacterial activity and mechanism of action of Monarda punctata essential oil and its main components against common bacterial pathogens in respiratory tract*. e-Century Publishing Corporation.

13 Swamy MK, MS Akhtar, and UR Sinniah. 2016. "Antimicrobial Properties of Plant Essential Oils against Human Pathogens and Their Mode of Action: An Updated Review". *Evidence-Based Complementary and Alternative Medicine*: ECAM. 2016.

14 Price, Shirley, and Len Price. 2015. *Aromatherapy for health professionals.* Edinburgh [etc.]: Churchill Livingstone. 76-79

15 Ibid

Chapter 20:
Polio

Polio is an alarming condition for parents to consider because of its ability to cause paralysis in children. The good news in the United States is that no cases of wild-type (occurring naturally) polio have originated since 1979. The last imported case was said to come into the United States in 1993.[1]

As of 2015, "eight countries reported cases of polio: Afghanistan, Equatorial Guinea, Lao People's Democratic Republic, Madagascar, Myanmar, Nigeria, Pakistan and Ukraine."[2] The Western hemisphere has been certified as free of indigenous wild poliovirus" since 1994.[3] More recently, as of 2005, a circulating vaccine-derived poliovirus (VDPV) has been identified in areas where under-vaccination occurs like the Amish community in the US.[4]

There are three serotypes of poliovirus that spread through respiratory routes or through fecal-oral route, for example, when changing the soiled diaper of a baby vaccinated with the live polio vaccine (which is not used in US but is still in use in other countries). Of the three types, type 2 was considered eradicated since 1999 and no new cases of type 3 have been reported since the last case in Nigeria in 2012.[5]

The large majority of cases of polio are asymptomatic (approximately 70% of infections). These people will have permanent immunity. People exposed to the virus with a mild infection will also have permanent immunity. Paralytic polio sometimes follows the initial infection or starts suddenly with paralysis coming on within 2–4 days of the onset of symptoms. In severe cases, if respiratory muscles become involved it can lead to a need for aggressive intervention and can be fatal.[6, 7] For unvaccinated children, risk factors that exist with poliovirus include traveling to other countries that still have cases of the active disease or use the live oral vaccine.

One of the strongest protective factors for polio is breastfeeding since mothers pass on antibodies that protect babies from many viruses and bacteria.[8]

Polio starts with the symptoms of the common cold and/or flu (fever, sore throat, headache, nausea/vomiting, fatigue, back and/or neck pain/

stiffness). If successfully treated in the early stages, it has a much reduced chance of developing into the more complicated symptom picture of paralysis (less than 1% of infected persons develops complications[9]).

Those that are more susceptible include people who are poorly nourished and, in general, are less well. For some people infected with the poliovirus, there may be no symptoms at all. If symptoms are present, they often last only 2–3 days. However, an infected person can transmit the virus for over two weeks through respiratory droplets and up to six weeks in the stool.

There is no conventional medical treatment for polio. Medical doctors may give pain relieving medications if necessary and promote range of motion exercises to maintain existing muscle tone. If respiratory muscles are affected, they will give oxygen to people who need it.

Vitalistic Naturopathic Approach

Basic naturopathic support includes bed rest, broths, oxymel, vitamin A, C and D, zinc, ginger tea, probiotics, garlic or magic socks, medicinal baths, hydrotherapy, dry skin brushing, lymphatic massage, steam inhalation, mushrooms and NAC. If you haven't already reviewed Part 3, that is the section where we discuss these therapies at length. The following suggestions are specific for working with polio.

Herbs

Early stage with cold/ flu symptoms:

- Antiviral herbs (viral meningitis) such as elderberry (*Sambucus nigra*), astragalus (*Astragalus membranaceus*), echinacea (*Echinacea angustifolia* and/or *Echinacea purpurea*), osha (*Ligusticum porteri*) can be consumed as glycerites.

- Antibacterial herbs such as goldenseal (*Hydrastis canadensis*), barberry (*Berberis vulgaris*), Oregon grape root (*Mahonia aquifolium*), coptis (*Coptis chinensis*). Because of their taste, they are best consumed as glycerites.

- Garlic or garlic and ginger oxymel to boost and support immune function.

- Osha (*Ligusticum porteri*) to help support immune and respiratory function.

Later stage with neurological symptoms:

- Milky oats (*Avena sativa*), linden tree (*Tilia europa*), gotu kola/ Indian pennywort (*Centella asiatica*) are known to support the nervous system.

- Licorice (*Glycyrrhiza glabra*) is an adaptogen (restores normal function), anti-inflammatory, antioxidant and reduces spasm. It is especially helpful for long-standing illness.

Supplements

- Early stage: vitamins A, C and D and zinc for immune support.

- Late stage: B12 chewable or drops, essential fatty acids, lecithin (sunflower based) or phosphatidylcholine (considerations here are that it's hard to find a non-soy based lecithin supplement and the phosphatidylcholine is the component of the lecithin that is supportive to brain cell membranes), d-ribose (for muscle energy), and carnosine[10] (for muscle recovery).

- Vitamin A flush: This is a treatment that can be highly effective but should be done under the supervision of a naturopathic physician or other qualified health care practitioner.

Essential Oils

- Pimento, one of the only essential oils known to directly affect the polio virus, is commonly known as Allspice (*Pimenta dioica*)[11]

- Roman chamomile (*Anthemis nobilis*) helps to reduce muscle spasms.[12]

- Combination to reduce spasms: two drops pimento and one drop Roman chamomile in one teaspoon of pure, organic vegetable oil. Massage into feet, legs, and arms 3-4 times a day.

Homeopathy

A child with polio will likely have common cold and/or flu symptoms of fever, sore throat, headache, nausea/vomiting, fatigue, back and/or neck pain and stiffness. The remedies listed here describe additional unique symptoms your child may have.

The easiest way to choose the remedy you think may work is to compare the list of symptoms you have made for your child to those listed under each remedy. Pick the one that seems to be the best match. For more explanation on how to create a list of symptoms, refer to the homeopathy section in Part 2 of this book.

When it comes to using homeopathic remedies for polio, Lathyrus sativus is discussed in the literature as one of the remedies that most closely matches the later, more complicated symptom picture of polio. However, when Polio was at it height in the early 20th century, Lath was used extensively both as a preventative remedy as well as a treatment, with great success. People who were given Lath rarely progressed past the early cold/flu symptom picture and those that did develop complications recovered with no further issue.

- ♦ The first remedies to consider in the early stages are those remedies discussed in the Hib section.

- ♦ **Lathyrus Sativus (Lath) 30C:**

  Used in the homeopathic prophylactic protocol to help reduce the risk and severity of symptoms.

  If considering Lath as a remedy to treat symptoms instead of as the homeopathic prophylactic, you would be looking for the following: spastic paralysis, infantile paralysis, paralysis which affects the lower extremities, heaviness, much weakness and slow recovery of nerve power. There may be excessive rigidity of the legs. The child may not be able to stretch out or cross the legs while sitting but can easily sit or bend forwards. The child may straighten up only with much difficulty. The skin may be very sensitive to touch, the legs blue, cold or burning and they may become swollen if they hang down. The tips of the fingers may be numb. There may be trembling, tottering or a rigid walk with a foot dragging (spastic gait) and the knees may knock against each other while walking. The reflexes are increased as compared to Cur in which they are decreased.

- ♦ **Conium (Con) 30C**

  There is a weakness and tingling sensation in the lower limbs which ascends to the upper part of the body and often starts with weakness in the legs and difficulty in walking. This initial complaint is followed by the symptoms spreading upwards.

The paralysis gradually progresses and can significantly affect breathing. This remedy covers painless paralytic conditions. There can also be a weakness of the muscles of the face and upper eyelids. The paralysis is often accompanied by numbness. There can be vertigo when turning the eyes, lying down or when looking at moving objects.

- **Curare (Cur) 30C**

  This remedy is all about paralysis and if this symptom is not present, it is hard to choose this remedy. There is a muscular paralysis, paralysis of the respiratory muscles and reflexes are diminished or absent (a characteristic symptom). Paralysis of the lower limbs starts with heaviness followed by stiffness, pain, weakness and difficulty walking. Symptoms are worse with movement, walking and ascending (e.g. climbing stairs). The legs tremble and give way in walking. There is facial paralysis, especially the left side, and paralysis of the tongue which is pulled to the right. This remedy is often used in the most rare presentations of polio that seem to primarily affect the face, eyes, tongue and respiratory nerves.

- **Gelsemium sempervirens (Gels) 30C**

  In Gels, the predominant symptoms are weakness, heaviness in the limbs and eyelids and chills running up and down back. There is often pain at the back of the neck with a heaviness of the head. Paralysis can be seen in all organs, limbs and the respiratory system. There is less rigidity of the muscles than is seen with Lath, rather the child is weak, trembles and has twitching in the muscles. The child may answer questions slowly or appear to be thinking slowly. There may be complaints of a bruised or sore sensation throughout the body. Often, the child is completely thirstless.

  - For homeopathic practitioners, in addition to the above mentioned remedies, the following ones have been written about in the literature as being more frequently indicated for paralytic states in general.[13]

  - Acon., Agar., Alum., Anac., Arg-n., Ars., Art-v., Bapt., Bar-c., Bell., Bry., Bufo, Calc., Calc-s., Caust., Cic., Chin., Cocc., Colch., Con., Crot-c., Crot-h., Cupr., Cur., Dros., Dulc.,

Gels., Kali-c., Kali-p., Kalm., Lath., Lach., Naja, Nat-m., Nit-ac., Nux-v., Old., Op., Phos., Plb., Rhus-t., Ruta, Sep., Sil., Stram., Sulph., Tarent., Verat., Zinc."

+ For the acute, infective and toxic forms of paralysis including infantile paralysis, a much narrower group of twenty-two remedies should be studied. Acon., Agar., Ars., Bell., Caust., Cocc., Cur., Dulc., Gels., Kali-p., Kalm., Lath., Lach., Naja., Nat-m., Nux-v., Op., Phos., Plb., Rhus-t., Stram., Zinc.

+ For cases that have passed the acute stage and end in chronic paralysis, the following thirteen remedies should be studied. Alum., Bar-c., Calc-s., Caust., Con., Cupr., Kali-p., Nat-m., Phos., Plb., Sil., Sulph., Zinc."

Other Therapies

The following therapies can be used to support healing from this condition.

Early Stages

+ Constitutional hydrotherapy to stimulate overall healing within the body and boost immune function.

+ Iodine rub to support local immune function.

Late Stages

+ Constitutional hydrotherapy for full body support.

+ Physical medicine: there are different types of physical therapies that can be supportive. Gentle massage and range of motion exercise can relieve muscle pain, maintain muscle tone and keep the body in proper alignment. Traditional physical therapy and craniosacral are supportive therapies to the nervous system.

1 Centers for Disease Control and Prevention. "Epidemiology and Prevention of Vaccine-Preventable Diseases Poliomyelitis." cdc.gov. https://www.cdc.gov/vaccines/pubs/pinkbook/polio.html (accessed February 1, 2017).

2 Centers for Disease Control and Prevention. "Global Health Polio Elimination in the United States For Healthcare Professionals." cdc.gov. https://www.cdc.gov/polio/us/hcp.html (accessed February 1, 2017).

3 Wallace, MD, MS, MPH, Gregory S., M. Steven Oberste, PhD. "Manual for the Surveillance of Vaccine-Preventable Diseases Chapter 12: Poliomyelitis." cdc.gov. https://www.cdc.gov/vaccines/pubs/surv-manual/chpt12-polio.html (accessed February 1, 2017).

4 Ibid

5 World Health Organization. "Poliomyelitis." who.int. http://www.who.int/mediacentre/factsheets/fs114/en/ (accessed February 1, 2017).

6 Centers for Disease Control and Prevention. "Global Health What Is Polio?" cdc.gov. https://www.cdc.gov/polio/about/ (accessed February 1, 2017).

7 Wallace, MD, MS, MPH, Gregory S., M. Steven Oberste, PhD. "Manual for the Surveillance of Vaccine-Preventable Diseases Chapter 12: Poliomyelitis." cdc.gov. https://www.cdc.gov/vaccines/pubs/surv-manual/chpt12-polio.html (accessed February 1, 2017).

8 Cerini, C., and G. M. Aldrovandi. 2013. "Breast milk: proactive immunomodulation and mucosal protection against viruses and other pathogens". *FUTURE VIROLOGY.* 8 (11): 1127-1134.

9 Centers for Disease Control and Prevention. "Epidemiology and Prevention of Vaccine-Preventable Diseases Poliomyelitis." cdc.gov. https://www.cdc.gov/vaccines/pubs/pinkbook/polio.html (accessed February 1, 2017).

10 Culbertson JY, RB Kreider, M Greenwood, and M Cooke. 2010. "Effects of beta-alanine on muscle carnosine and exercise performance: a review of the current literature". *Nutrients.* 2 (1): 75-98.

11 Price, Shirley, and Len Price. 2015. *Aromatherapy for health professionals.* Edinburgh [etc.]: Churchill Livingstone. 90-91

12 Schnaubelt, Kurt. 1998. *Advanced aromatherapy: the science of essential oil therapy.* Rochester, Vt: Healing Arts Press. 64

13 Grimmer, Arthur Hill, and Ahmed Currim. 1996. *The collected works of Arthur Hill Grimmer M.D.* Norwalk, Conn: Hahnemann International Institute for Homeopathic Documentation.

Chapter 21:
Rubella (German Measles)

Rubella has been considered eradicated in the US since 2004.[1] Today less than ten cases per year are reported in the US. Most of those cases are usually imported. The WHO is currently working on worldwide eradication programs.

Rubella is a contagious togavirus of the Rubivirus genus. It is an enveloped RNA virus that is relatively unstable and is inactivated by items such as lipid solvents, ultraviolet light, heat, low pH and trypsin. Rubella is transmitted via respiratory droplets and enters the body through the respiratory tract, especially the nose and throat. Infections primarily occur in late winter and early spring.

Symptoms of rubella infection are usually mild. Children will initially display a rash that can be itchy, but isn't always. The rash can be pale or bright red and travels from the face to the rest of body. It fades so quickly that a child's face may be clear by the time the rash starts to show up on his or her extremities. The rash lasts about three days. Within a couple of days of the rash appearing, it will be accompanied by a slight fever, headache, mild conjunctivitis, cough, runny nose and slight enlargement of the superficial glands of the neck and behind the ears. Up to 50% of people show no symptoms.[2, 3] The entire duration of illness is usually 5–7 days. Risks and complications of rubella for children are rare. They include thrombocytopenic purpura and encephalitis.[4]

When rubella resembles rubeola, there is a discrete, maculopapular rash of pale red color, the eruptive points being slightly elevated and about the size of a pin's head or larger. These lesions have a tendency to come together upon the face, particularly when they are numerous.

When rubella resembles scarlatina, the rash is of a diffuse, uniform, scarlet color, but is never as intense, however, as in scarlet fever. The maculopapular rash occurs on the forehead, fingers and toes and about the wrists.

There may be some desquamation (peeling off of skin) after the rash resolves. There may or may not be catarrhal symptoms and throat symptoms may be so slight they go unnoticed. There may be a slight cough present. The superficial cervical axillary and inguinal lymph glands may or may not be swollen, although this is one of the characteristic symptoms of the disease.

To date, there is no conventional medical treatment available for rubella.

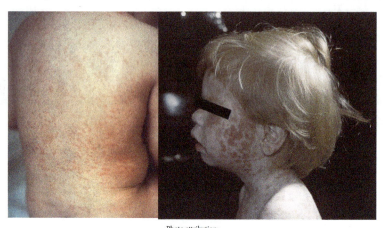

Photo attribution:
By CDC - crop of File:Rash of rubella on skin of child's back.JPG, Public Domain, https://commons.wikimedia.org/w/index.php?curid=39884727
By CDC - http://phil.cdc.gov/phil/details.asp, Public Domain, https://commons.wikimedia.org/w/index.php?curid=40409843

Vitalistic Naturopathic Approach

Basic naturopathic support includes bed rest, broths, oxymel, vitamin A, C and D, zinc, ginger tea, probiotics, garlic or magic socks, medicinal baths, hydrotherapy, dry skin brushing, lymphatic massage, steam inhalation, mushrooms and NAC. If you haven't already reviewed Part 3, that is the section where we discuss these therapies at length. To keep a child with rubella comfortable, topical ointments for itching and tepid sponge baths can be helpful as well. The following suggestions are specific for working with rubella.

Herbs

- Nettles (*Urtica dioica*) as a tea or glycerite soothes itchiness.

- Lemon balm (*Melissa officinalis*) as a tea or glycerite acts as a mild pain reliever, has antiviral effects, eases anxiety by calming the nervous system. In some cases, it can act as a sedative.

- Burdock (*Arctium lappa*) as a tea or a base for a soup, it helps skin recover and heal more quickly.

- Antiviral herbs (viral meningitis) such as elderberry (*Sambucus nigra*), astragalus (*Astragalus membranaceus*), echinacea (*Echinacea angustifolia* and/or *Echinacea purpurea*), osha (*Ligusticum porteri*) can be consumed as glycerites.

Supplements

Vitamin A flush: This is a treatment that can be highly effective but should be done under the supervision of a naturopathic physician or other qualified health care practitioner.

Essential Oils

Essential oils can help address the underlying viral infection that causes German measles as well as soothe the itching.

- *Ravensara aromatica* has strong antiviral activity.[5]

- German chamomile (*Matricaria chamomilla*) soothes skin irritation and itching.

- Tea tree (*Melaleuca alternifolia*) also has antiviral effects and is helpful to soothe any skin irritation.

- Lavender (*Lavandula angustifolia*) soothes the skin, reduces itching, and has mild antiviral effects. Lavender also has a calming effect which can be very helpful for children suffering with itching and other symptoms.

  - You can use this combination of three essential oils in the bath:

  - Two drops each of ravensara, German chamomile (or lavender), and tea tree essential oil to one tablespoon of milk (cow, goat, almond, coconut, hemp, etc.) The oil and protein in the milk helps to disperse the essential oil in the bathwater. Avoid adding essential oils directly to the bathwater. They do not disperse and can cause skin irritation.

- Add to a warm bath and soak as long as desired.

- Create an oil to rub into the skin. If you are an adult applying the oil to a child's skin, use latex-free gloves to avoid contaminating yourself and others.

- Add two drops of ravensara, German chamomile, and tea tree essential oils to a tablespoon of pure, organic vegetable oil. Rub into the skin 3–4 times a day. Rub the oil first into the soles of the feet; then into the affected areas.

- For children under six years old, dilute the essential oils in two tablespoons of pure, organic vegetable oil.

Homeopathy

A child with rubella will first often have a rash that may or may not be itchy. The rash can be pale or bright red and travels from the face to the rest of body. It fades so quickly that a child's face may be clear by the time the rash starts to show up on other parts of the body. The rash lasts about three days and just before it begins to clear, there may be symptoms of slight fever, headache, mild conjunctivitis, cough, runny nose and slight enlargement of the glands on the neck and behind the ears. But, up to 50% of children show no symptoms at all. The remedies listed here describe additional unique symptoms your child may have.

The easiest way to choose the remedy you think may work is to compare the list of symptoms you have made for your child to those listed under each remedy. Pick the one that seems to be the best match. For more explanation on how to create a list of symptoms, refer to the homeopathy section in Part 2 of this book.

The following remedies are the most common for this condition but keep in mind that the best remedy for your child may not be listed here. If you're having difficulty choosing a remedy, consider working with a homeopathic or naturopathic doctor to choose the best remedy.

- **Rubeola (Rubeol) 30C:**

  used in the homeopathic prophylactic protocol to help reduce the risk and severity of symptoms.

- **Aconitum napellus (Acon) 30C**

  Like with Bell there is a rapid onset of symptoms. Often there is fever, chilliness and restlessness or fear. The face may be red or pale in color and the pulse is often rapid. If there is a cough, it is short, dry and intense with a loud and sharp quality. The cough is typically worse at night, in general, especially around midnight. The child feels better and the cough is better in the open air, however, the onset may have followed an exposure to cold air. The rash may not be present or may be slow to develop and not widespread. Often the child's skin is hot and the rash may itch.

◆ **Belladonna (Bell) 30C**

The symptoms start suddenly. The face or head may hot but the hands and feet are cold. The skin is red. The eyes can be glazed and the pupils dilated. The child will complain of head or muscle pain and if they can communicate the kind of pain it will be a throbbing or pounding sensation. Like we see in Bry, all pains are worse with motion and jarring or bumped. They are over-sensitive to light, noise and being touched. The symptoms are typically worse at 3 PM. They are not very thirsty. The rash is usually bright red, appears sudden and travels quickly to the other parts of the body. It disappears from the face as suddenly as it appeared.

◆ **Bryonia alba (Bry) 30C**

When Bry is indicated, you will see the child want to lie still and not be bothered. If there is a cough it will be a dry cough which hurts the head and chest and the child may hold the chest when coughing. The lips are dry and the tongue is coated. There is a great thirst for large quantities of water at long intervals. The rash can be slow to appear but once established it is widespread but may suddenly disappear.

◆ **Gelsemium sempervirens (Gels) 30C**

The symptoms come on slowly. There is usually a slowly developing fever and headache which starts at the back of the head and which spreads to the forehead. There is a sense of heaviness in the head and the eyes feel heavy or the eyelids look part-way closed. The child looks drowsy. They are not thirsty, even with a fever, and may have chills, especially along the spine. They may also have trembling and complain of weakness. The rash will be very itchy and bright or dark red.

◆ **Pulsatilla pratensis (Puls) 30C**

In Puls, the rash can be slow to come out and when it does it is more dark red than bright red. The spots may have pus. The skin is itchy and worse with heat and better in a cool bath or with cool rags. This child is often thirstless and can be very clingy and weepy. Being in a closed, warm room will worsen their symptoms while being in cool, open air will help them feel better. The fever is usually low-grade. This child may have a very dry mouth and frequently lick their lips but they will not ask for something to drink.

Other Therapies

The following therapies can be used to support healing from this condition.

- Burdock (*Arctium lappa*) poultice to soothe the skin.

- Calendula (*Calendula officinalis*) wash to soothe the skin and promote healing.

- Soaking bath drawn with baking soda, cornstarch or oats to soothe the skin

- Aloe vera gel, chickweed (*Stellaria media*) poultice, lavender (*Lavandula spp.*) poultice or oil topically soothe the skin.

1 Centers for Disease Control and Prevention. "Rubella (German Measles, Three-Day Measles) Rubella in the U.S.." cdc.gov. https://www.cdc.gov/rubella/about/in-the-us.html (accessed February 1, 2017).

2 Centers for Disease Control and Prevention. "Rubella (German Measles, Three-Day Measles) Signs and Symptoms." cdc.gov. https://www.cdc.gov/rubella/about/symptoms.html (accessed February 1, 2017).

3 Centers for Disease Control and Prevention. "Epidemiology and Prevention of Vaccine-Preventable Diseases Rubella." cdc.gov. https://www.cdc.gov/vaccines/pubs/pinkbook/rubella.html#epi (accessed February 1, 2017).

4 Centers for Disease Control and Prevention. "Rubella (German Measles, Three-Day Measles) For Healthcare Professionals." cdc.gov. https://www.cdc.gov/rubella/hcp.html (accessed February 1, 2017).

5 Price, Shirley, and Len Price. 2015. *Aromatherapy for health professionals.* Edinburgh [etc.]: Churchill Livingstone. 90-91

Chapter 22:
Rotavirus

Rotavirus is an intestinal virus that affects infants and children around the world. It is so common in the US the CDC estimates that by age five all children will have had rotavirus at least once.[1] It is linked to cases of diarrhea with accompanying cramping, fever and possible vomiting. It has an incubation period of 1–3 days and usually resolves in about a week. There is a seasonality associated with it showing a prevalence occurring in the winter and spring from December to May in the US. It is resistant to antibacterial soap and common disinfectants, making routine handwashing an important route for prevention. It is contagious and transmitted from personal contact primarily via the fecal-oral route or through contact with contaminated objects, and can be ingested through contaminated water or food.[2] Risk factors for infants and small children are being in daycare settings and swimming in public pools.

Current data as of June 2017, shows that one in 20,000 children become infected. Children less than five years old are the largest group affected with infants less than one year old more severely affected.[3] The CDC states that as many as 20–60 deaths occur annually in the US.[4] The biggest risk and complication connected to it is dehydration, which can lead to electrolyte imbalance and death if not addressed.

One of the vaccines available for it has been on and off the market over the last thirteen years due to cases of intussusception (bowels folding in on themselves leading to life threatening bowel obstruction) connected to the vaccine. The latest version of the vaccine has not caused as many cases of intussusception but it is still listed as a possible side effect. Interestingly, the CDC does not recommend initiating vaccination for rotavirus if a child is older than fifteen weeks of age.[5]

With rotavirus, it is an issue of when, not if, a child will be exposed to it. Hydration is the most important item to be aware of when children have diarrhea whether or not it's caused by rotavirus. Oftentimes, children have diarrhea and parents don't know what caused it. It's possible that rotavirus was behind it but parents do not run to the doctor for every case of diarrhea. They usually do normal care at home and allow the body to resolve the diarrhea on its own.

Symptoms of a rotavirus infection can develop within forty-eight hours of exposure to the virus and include fever, nausea, and vomiting, abdominal cramps and frequent, watery, foul and sometimes bloody diarrhea. There may also be a cough, runny nose, thirst, irritability, restlessness, lethargy, sunken eyes, a dry mouth and tongue, dry skin, decreased urination and, in infants, a dry diaper for several hours. As with all viral infections, there may be few or no symptoms. Rotavirus usually resolves within ten days.

The conventional medical world does not have a treatment for rotavirus infection. Doctors may give IV fluids if diarrhea has been severe. However, in most cases, they wait for the body to resolve the infection on its own. For children that are breastfed, breastmilk is considered protective.

A Vitalistic Naturopathic Approach

Basic naturopathic support includes bed rest, broths, oxymel, vitamin A, C and D, zinc, ginger tea, probiotics, garlic or magic socks, medicinal baths, hydrotherapy, dry skin brushing, lymphatic massage, steam inhalation, mushrooms and NAC. If you haven't already reviewed Part 3, that is the section where we discuss these therapies at length.

A potential serious complication because of the diarrhea is dehydration. There are many ways to keep your little one hydrated including flavoring water with a bit of fruit, electrolyte drinks, frozen, healthy homemade treats. The following suggestions are specific for working with rotavirus.

Herbs

- Elderberry (*Sambucus nigra*) is best taken as a syrup or glycerite. It is a general immune tonic increasing white blood cell activity and has antimicrobial effects.

- Astragalus (*Astragalus membranaceus*) is best taken as a syrup or glycerite. It is an adaptogenic herb which restores normal function, has anti-inflammatory and antiviral effects and is an immunomodulator.

- Echinacea (*Echinacea angustifolia* and/or *Echinacea purpurea*) an antimicrobial herb best used as a glycerite which is supportive for the immune system.

- Ginger (*Zingiber officinalis*) or ginger and thyme (*Thymus vulgaris*) as a tea. Together the ginger can address nausea, vomiting and ease pain while thyme can act as an antiviral herb.

Supplements

+ Vitamin A flush: This is a treatment that can be highly effective but should be done under the supervision of a Naturopathic Physician or other qualified health care practitioner.

Caution: Vitamin C and Magnesium can stimulate the bowels, worsening diarrhea.

Essential Oils

Research shows that carvacrol, a specific constituent found in several essential oils, inhibits rotavirus.[6] Although Mexican oregano contains carvacrol, the whole essential oil does not inhibit rotavirus as effectively as carvacrol alone.

Carvacrol is highest in thyme essential oil, particularly the chemotype carvacrol. Look for "Thyme ct carvacrol." Ideally the oil will be distilled from plants harvested in the autumn, when carvacrol content is at its highest level.

Keep in mind that thyme essential oil is very caustic and must be diluted in vegetable oil (safflower or sunflower oil are ideal). Dilute the essential oil and rub into the abdomen 3–4 times a day.

+ Infants: one drop of thyme ct carvacrol essential oil in two tablespoons of vegetable oil.

+ 18 months-6 years old: one drop of thyme ct carvacrol essential oil in four tablespoons of vegetable oil

+ 6–12 years old: one drop thyme ct carvacrol in two teaspoons of vegetable oil

To reduce the cramping associated with diarrhea, add one drop of Roman chamomile (Chamaemelum nobile/Anthemis nobilis) to the above mixture. Rub into the abdomen 3–4 times a day.

Homeopathy

A child with rotavirus will likely have a fever, nausea and vomiting, abdominal cramps and frequent, watery, foul and sometimes bloody diarrhea. There may also be a cough, runny nose, thirst, irritability, restlessness, lethargy, sunken eyes, a dry mouth and tongue, dry skin, decreased urination and, in infants, a dry diaper for several hours. The remedies listed here describe additional unique symptoms your child may have.

The easiest way to choose the remedy you think may work is to compare the list of symptoms you have made for your child to those listed under each remedy. Pick the one that seems to be the best match. For more explanation on how to create a list of symptoms, refer to the homeopathy section in Part 2 of this book.

The following remedies are the most common for this condition but keep in mind that the best remedy for your child may not be listed here. If you're having difficulty choosing a remedy, consider working with a homeopathic or naturopathic doctor to choose the best remedy.

- ◆ **Rota (Rota) 30C:**

    Used in the homeopathic prophylactic protocol to help reduce the risk and severity of symptoms.

- ◆ **Arsenicum album (Ars) 30C**

    This may be one of the most effective remedies, if the symptom picture matches, for the developed rotavirus infection. There are large quantities of diarrhea and vomiting which may happen at the same time and appear after eating and drinking. There can be pains, cramping and/or a burning sensation in the abdomen at any point but also just before the vomiting and/or diarrhea. The child will usually be quite thirsty but only sips water in small amounts and prefers it to be cold. Warm drinks, while not preferred, may help improve the symptoms temporarily. There is usually some weakness or exhaustion that follows the diarrhea, but, on the other hand, there may be some restlessness, especially of the mind and the child may be anxious. Fever with chills can be present and the child will typically be chilly and sensitive to and worse from the cold. The stools can be varied in Ars but are often bloody, slimy or offensive. In rotavirus infection, the diarrhea is more prevalent than the vomiting.

- **China (Chin) 30C (also called Cinchona)**

  The child's diarrhea is often accompanied by extreme exhaustion, bloating and excessive gas. They feel exhausted, weak and even sleepy. Fainting spells may be present. The symptoms are worse at night, in hot weather and after nursing. Abdominal pain, often on the right side in the area of the liver, is much better when they bend over. The abdominal pains may also be better for a short period of time after they pass stool. There is typically a great deal of irritability. The fever may not start until after diarrhea starts. The stool is frothy, yellow (sometimes bloody with rotavirus infection), painless and often accompanied by passing of gas.

- **Podophyllum (Podo) 30C**

  There is typically gushing, large amounts of diarrhea which may be bloody or greenish and watery. The stool is often quite foul and may contain particles of undigested food or yellow globules. There is often a sudden urgency for stool that may drive the child out of bed early in the morning or in younger children may cause them to have an accident. There is often significant rumbling and gurgling in the abdomen just before the stool. Between stools there is cramping in the abdomen, often severe enough to cause the child to bend over in pain. Frequently, passing the stool is painless. Often there is a great thirst for cold drinks.

- **Veratrum Album (Verat) 30C**

  With Verat, dehydration is a key symptom. The stool is watery, comes out in a forcible stream and is accompanied by pain and cramping in abdomen. Abdominal pain may precede the stool. The child may complain of a cold feeling in abdomen which may be swollen and painful to touch. There is often vomiting and the vomiting and diarrhea may happen at the same time as with Ars. However, this child will be cold, sweaty and incredibly weak. The body gets cold and breaks into a cold sweat, all over but especially on the head. There is a craving for ice and cold drinks.

  - Other remedies to consider as reported in the literature: Aloe, Phos, Crot, Merc, Merc-c, Nux-v, Nat-m, Colch, Ham.

Other Therapies

The following therapies can be used to support healing from this condition.

- Homemade Electrolyte drink maintains hydration. (This is very important!) Add ½ teaspoon raw sugar and a pinch of sea salt, Himalayan salt or mineral salt in 8 ounces of filtered water.

- Coconut water in small amounts due to its high sugar content.

- Dietary adjustments: add potatoes and bananas to the diet as they can bind up stool. Bieler's broth can help restore hydration.

- Medicinal bath with lavender essential oil to calm a restless child.

- Breastfeeding will maintain hydration. If a child is breastfeeding, continue breastfeeding as usual.

1 Centers for Disease Control and Prevention. "Rotavirus Clinical Information." cdc.gov. https://www.cdc.gov/rotavirus/clinical.html (accessed February 1, 2017).

2 Ibid

3 Ibid

4 Payne PhD, MSPH, Daniel C., Mary Wikswo, MPH, and Umesh D. Parashar, MBBS, MPH. "Manual for the Surveillance of Vaccine-Preventable Diseases Chapter 13." cdc.gov. https://www.cdc.gov/vaccines/pubs/surv-manual/ chpt13-rotavirus.html (accessed February 1, 2017).

5 Centers for Disease Control and Prevention. "Recommended Immunization Schedule for Children and Adolescents Aged 18 Years or Younger, UNITED STATES, 2017." cdc.gov. https://www.cdc.gov/vaccines/schedules/downloads/ child/0-18yrs-child-combined-schedule.pdf (accessed February 1, 2017).

6 Alves, Sydney Hartz, Sandra Arenhart, Ana Paula Cueto, Luciane Teresinha Lovato, Marciele Ribas Pilau, and Rudi Weiblen. 2011. "Antiviral activity of the Lippia graveolens (Mexican oregano) essential oil and its main compound carvacrol against human and animal viruses". *Brazilian Journal of Microbiology.* 42 (4): 1616-1624.

Chapter 23:
Tetanus

Tetanus is an infection caused by the anaerobic bacteria *Clostridium tetani*. It can infect a person through a puncture wound with an item that had the bacteria on it. Historically, people came across it living on farms because the bacteria lives in the intestines of cattle, sheep and small animals like guinea pigs, rats, cats and dogs. It is found in the manure of horses and other farm animals.

Rates of tetanus infection have consistently dropped since the year 1900 as more people started living in cities and have had less contact with farm animals. Today, a wound can become infected if it is exposed to contaminated feces or dead tissue. The most up-to-date number of people affected is from 2009 with nineteen cases reported to the CDC and two deaths in the US[1] Data from the CDC show that the greatest number of people affected were over sixty-five years old. Of those people nearly ⅓ of them were diabetic or IV drug users. Tetanus is not contagious.

Tetanus is concerning to the medical community because it causes a sudden and involuntary tightening of muscles that can happen anywhere in the body. The most notable symptom was known as lockjaw because a person's mouth would remain locked in a contracted position. It became problematic if it caused contraction of the diaphragm because it would not allow the muscles needed for respiration to contract and relax normally.

The incubation period for tetanus ranges from 2–16 days and many times the person does not even remember the injury. One of the early symptoms is a sore throat with painful swallowing. This can lead to symptoms of rigidity either in the area of the injury or in one part of the body. This can spread to become what is known as generalized tetanus (muscle rigidity) and trismus (lockjaw). Whether it is localized or general tetanus, other symptoms can include muscle stiffness, neck stiffness, restlessness, and spasmodic reflexes.

In the late stage, the muscle rigidity becomes the major symptom. This rigidity spreads downward from the jaw and facial muscles to the extensor muscles of the limbs. The spasms last seconds to minutes and become more frequent and intense as the condition progresses. There can be difficulty breathing and rapid heart rate or increased blood pressure. The contraction of the face muscles over a period of time is what produces the frozen grin, also known as risus sardonicus. This is usually a clinical diagnosis as there is no specific diagnostic laboratory test.

If a child were to become infected with *C. tetani*, medical doctors will give antibiotics, a tetanus immunoglobulin shot (an antitoxin) and the tetanus vaccine.. Their aim is to clean out any wound and keep the muscles relaxed, which might also prompt them to prescribe muscle relaxers.

A Vitalistic Naturopathic Approach

At home, wound cleaning is the first step to take with any kind of puncture would. Items like hydrogen peroxide can clean out a wound with minimal discomfort (while cleaning out a wound with alcohol can have a child screaming in no time).

Other natural approaches include increasing immune functioning with nutrients like vitamin C and using antimicrobial herbs like Oregon grape root (*Mahonia aquifolium*) to help fight off infections. Increasing probiotics adds extra beneficial microorganisms to keep a child's body functioning well. Using alternating hydrotherapy treatments increases white blood production keeping the immune system primed.

Basic naturopathic support includes bed rest, broths, oxymel, vitamin A, C and D, zinc, ginger tea, probiotics, garlic or magic socks, medicinal baths, hydrotherapy, dry skin brushing, lymphatic massage, steam inhalation, mushrooms and NAC. If you haven't already reviewed Part 3, that is the section where we discuss these therapies at length. The following suggestions are specific for working with tetanus.

Herbs

- Berberine containing antibacterial herbs such as goldenseal (*Hydrastis canadensis*), barberry (*Berberis vulgaris*), Oregon grape root (*Mahonia aquifolium*), coptis (*Coptis chinensis*). Because of their taste, they are best consumed as glycerites. Although these are not discussed in botanical medical literature as being specific to tetanus, they are general antibacterial herbs. Choose one of these herbs.

- Licorice (*Glycyrrhiza glabra*) is an adaptogen (restores normal function), anti-inflammatory, antioxidant and reduces spasm. It is especially helpful for long-standing illness.

Supplements

♦ Magnesium glycinate is most easily used as a powder mixed in liquid such as water. It keeps muscles relaxed.

Essential Oils

♦ Immediately after washing the wound and dosing homeopathic Ledum, apply tea tree (*Melaleuca alternifolia*)[2] essential oil. Tea tree is one of the few essential oils that can be applied "neat," without dilution, although you may want to dilute with vegetable oil for a young child. If you are away from a water source and have tea tree essential oil, apply the oil as soon as possible and repeat applications of the oil every 20–30 minutes. Continue applying tea tree oil to the wound three times a day until all signs of infection have resolved.

Homeopathy

A child with tetanus may have a sore throat with painful swallowing and symptoms of rigidity either in general or in the area of the injury. They may also have muscle and neck stiffness, risus sardonicus, restlessness and spasmodic reflexes. In addition to these, you will notice that there are more specific qualities that may be unique to what your child is experiencing. The remedies listed here describe unique symptoms your child may have.

The easiest way to choose the remedy you think may work is to compare the list of symptoms you have made for your child to those listed under each remedy. Pick the one that seems to be the best match. For more explanation on how to create a list of symptoms, refer to the homeopathy section in Part 2 of this book.

The following remedies are the most common for this condition but keep in mind that the best remedy for your child may not be listed here. If you're having difficulty choosing a remedy, consider working with a homeopathic or naturopathic doctor to choose the best remedy.

♦ **Ledum (Led) 30C**

A classic homeopathic remedy used for puncture wounds. In fact, one of the great homeopaths, Dr. James Tyler Kent (1849–1916), said that one should give homeopathic Led as soon as possible after any puncture wound. Used in the homeopathic prophylactic protocol to help reduce the risk and severity of symptoms and after a concerning puncture wound. The wound may appear pale or white in the center surrounded by redness with a cooler temperature in the center than the surrounding skin. Conversely, there may be swelling and redness around the wound or a purple/white mottling color. Cold water or applications of ice tend to improve the symptoms. This is also called for in tetanus with twitching of the muscles near the wound.

◆ **Angustura (Ang) 30C**

There may be a sustained muscle contraction (tetanic) rigidity of the muscles and/or a painful stiffness and stretching of the limbs. The child's lips may be drawn back showing their teeth (risus sardonicus) and the jaws may be locked. You may observe spasmodic twitching or jerking of the muscles or trance or seizure with a loss of sensation and consciousness accompanied by rigidity of the body (catalepsy) with their body bent backward. Convulsions in general can be part of this remedy with twitching and jerking along the back, like electric shocks. Spasms, twitchings and convulsions, if present, are usually worse when the child is touched or if they drink lukewarm water.

◆ **Arsenicum album (Ars) 30C**

Convulsions may be present and have such a severe stiffness that no joint can be moved. Twitchings, cramps and tetanic spasms of the muscles are seen. The child may be hysterical and cannot be comforted or calmed down. This hysteria may include spasms or convulsions followed by exhaustion and unconsciousness. They may feel or become faint in the morning with purple lips, coldness of the extremities, anxiety, and prostration. Things that may make the symptoms better include hot bathing and hot drinks. A striking symptom of Ars is greatly increased levels of anxiety.

◆ **Belladonna (Bell) 30C**

The symptoms of Bell tend to come on very quickly and are fully developed. There may be a red flush to the skin or the child may complain of a throbbing and pounding pain.

The jaws may be very stiff. You may see much twitching and sudden startling to noises or movements. Often the child's eyes will have dilated pupils and they may just be staring off into pace. The convulsions of Bell can be severe. There may also be rigidity of the throat muscles, jerking of the limbs and severe tension of the body muscles. This remedy is indicated for tetanus in infants. Striking symptoms of this remedy include the sudden onset and the throbbing pains.

♦ **Camphora officinalis (Camph) 30C**

The tendency for convulsions and spasms in Camph is well known. Lockjaw and other tetanus symptoms are usually present. There may be twisting movements of the muscles and tendons (Subsultus tendinum) with excitability, jerking, twitching and trembling may be present. The arms may spasmodically move in circles (rotation). The head is often spasmodically drawn backward or to one side. The eyes are convulsively turned upward. Epileptic-like seizures are followed by a state of extreme exhaustion.

♦ **Cicuta virosa (Cic) 30C**

A useful homeopathic remedy in tetanic convulsions, with sudden rigidity and jerkings followed by prostration. The child may have great difficulty of breathing, lockjaw, arching back (opisthotonos) which is all worse when they are touched. There are spasms in the esophagus which may be identified by their inability to swallow something. A striking symptom is that they fix their eyes and stare at one thing in the room.

♦ **Gelsemium sempervirens (Gels) 30C**

The child may have paralysis of the pharynx, tongue, throat or lungs. The child may complain of feeling heavy or that it is difficult to lift his or her arms, legs or keep the eyes open. In fact, you may see that the eyelids appear to be half-closed. The child will complain of a chill that runs up and down the back. You may see trembling or shivering. The striking symptom is the paralysis.

♦ **Hydrocyanic acid (Hydr-ac) 30C**

There may be persistent sudden, abnormal, involuntary

muscular contraction consisting of a continued muscular
contraction (tonic spasm). may be present and is very common
in the muscles of the face, jaws and back. There is lockjaw
and risus sardonicus with difficult breathing. There may be a
bright, livid redness to the face with frothing at the mouth. The
body is rigid and bent backwards with an arched back. The
attack is sudden and the reflexes may be exaggerated but not as
much as with Strych.

+ **Hypericum (Hyper) 30C**

In this remedy, we can see lockjaw develop after an injury
to nerves. It is considered a prophylactic remedy in cases of
wounds of palms or soles and is especially useful in spinal
injuries.

+ **Nux vomica (Nux-v) 30C**

Nux-v is an important homeopathic remedy for tetanus. It
has tetanic convulsions with opisthotonos, difficult or painful
breathing. We often see the textbook picture of tetanus, with
its convulsion of muscles renewed by the slightest external
impression (touch, sound, smells, light), risus sardonicus,
respiratory spasm, blue discoloration of the face and a clear
mind.

+ **Physostigma (Phys) 30C**

With Phys, the sensory nerves are irritable and external
impressions worsen the child's symptoms. There are tetanic
spasms with stiffness of the spine and legs. The pupils alternate
between dilation and contraction. There may be sudden,
violent, involuntary contraction of the muscles of the body
and an inability to precisely control bodily movements. The
child may also complain of numbness in paralyzed parts and
cramping pains in limbs.

+ **Strychninum (Strych) 30C**

When this remedy is needed you may see sudden, violent,
involuntary contraction of the muscles of the body which
can be accompanied by loss of consciousness, but should be
especially thought of when the consciousness is retained.
There may be a distortion of the eyes that can appear as highly

congested and in constant motion, or red and protruding
or sunken and rolling. They may have the eyes and/or head
turned to one side of the face. There can be shortness of breath.
Any touch can trigger the spasms or other symptoms and they
are also worse from light or noise. Reflexes can be extremely
exaggerated, more so than in Hydr-ac.

- **Veratrum album (Verat) 30C**

  The child may have lockjaw with spasms of the glottis (the
  space between the vocal cords) and a constriction or tightness
  of the chest that feels like suffocation. The hands and feet are
  drawn inwards and the pupils are contracted.

Other Therapies

- Plantain (*Plantago major*) poultice applied externally to the
  wound. It is a soothing herb and helps draw out infection.

1 Tejpratap, S. P. and Tiwari MD. Centers for Disease Control and Prevention. "Manual for the Surveillance of Vaccine-Preventable Diseases, Chapter 16." cdc.gov. https://www.cdc.gov/vaccines/pubs/surv-manual/chpt16-tetanus. html (accessed February 1, 2017).

2 Price, Shirley, and Len Price. 2015. *Aromatherapy for health professionals.* Edinburgh [etc.]: Churchill Livingstone. 76

PART V:
Closing Thoughts

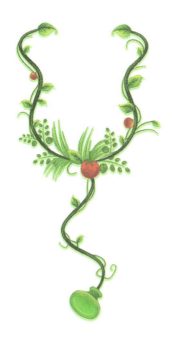

Dr. Camp's Closing Thoughts

Writing this book was very important to me personally for a number of reasons. First, in the course of working with people from all over the world who have made the decision not to vaccinate, I have inevitably faced many of the childhood illnesses. In the beginning, as a new practitioner, I struggled to find the information to treat from a vitalistic approach. The information and treatments used by previous generations of physicians who saw these illnesses on a regular basis and treated them successfully were buried in history. As I did research, dug through the old literature, learned from my naturopathic elders, compiled notes and saw incredible success, I knew that I needed to make this information available to everyone, parents and caregivers alike.

Second, as the truth about the pharmaceutical industry and particularly the vaccination program comes to light, and as more and more people choose not to vaccinate, it is imperative that all caregivers-parents, grandparents, doctors and other healthcare providers-have this knowledge. Armed with knowledge, we can safely and effectively nurse our children through conditions that have been around for thousands upon thousands of years. They come out on the other end with life-long immunity and no damage from vaccination. It is important to note here that most of these conditions are not life-threatening, as long as basic health is established and maintained.

Last, but not least, I want to discuss something with all of you that I routinely discuss with my mainstream (non-holistic) colleagues. Often, when they find out I have treated measles or mumps, they will exclaim with shock and sometimes dismay:"What! You did not get them on antibiotics? Do you know the dangers of untreated disease?" To which I calmly reply, "Well, I agree there are risks to untreated illness. But I am treating, just not with your therapies. I am treating with naturopathic therapies." So, stand strong in your decision, arm yourself with knowledge, partner with a vitalistic naturopathic doctor and above all, cherish those bright shining lights in your life. They grow up way, way too fast.

Dr. Thompson's Closing Thoughts

With so much information available today, parents can get confused about how to best care for their children. They struggle making decisions that are correct for their families. Whether or not they have vaccinated their children, they are being faced with a rise in contagious illnesses. They are concerned about vaccination side effects. Meanwhile, both arguments—either for vaccinating or not vaccinating—are strongly based on fear. Parents don't know what kinds of risks they might be taking if they go one way or the other. It shouldn't be this way. Parents should have complete information and understanding to make the best decisions for their families.

All parents want to take the best possible care of their children. Understanding the severity of childhood illnesses better prepares them to know how to handle different conditions. Providing parents with information that gives them confidence and knowing their children are being well cared for gives them peace of mind. This is invaluable in a country where fear-based decision-making is perpetuated by pharmaceutical companies. As I studied the conventional medicine treatments available for different childhood illness, I realized they were either nonexistent or were becoming ineffective (consider the rising rates of antibiotic resistance). Of course mainstream practitioners would push for vaccinations if the only treatment therapies they have are incapable of keeping children healthy. However, with side effects associated with vaccinations, they aren't a viable option for many parents.

The therapies provided throughout this book are ones I have personally seen, been mentored in by naturopathic elders or have researched and found to be effective. Some of these natural treatments go back well over a century, many of which were available before pharmaceutical drugs were around. This gives us historical precedence. As children grow and develop, it is our job to give them the best possibility of maturing into well-adjusted adults in every sense: physically, mentally, emotionally and spiritually. It is my sincere hope that parents looking for healthy options for childhood illnesses find this book a useful resource over many years.

PART VI:
The Apothecary

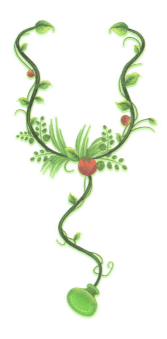

This section contains information on dosing, use and preparation of the herbs, supplements, supplies and other therapies discussed in this book. The majority of these items can be purchased in your local healthfood store or online. For some products that are not easily found, we listed suggestions in The Resources section.

Herbal Information

We have given herbal suggestions for all conditions in the Conditions section. It is not necessary, nor is it helpful, to use all the herbs listed to treat each condition. In fact, if the condition is bacterial in nature, only one or two of the antimicrobial herbs are necessary. We have indicated what symptoms each herb addresses, let this guide you in choosing herbs.

The part of the plant used and how much you dose are both important. This section guides you through the process of choosing proper plant parts and doses. In addition, dosing depends greatly on the age of your child and the herbal preparation you are using, so be sure to take those factors into account as well.

Herbalist Rosemary Gladstar explains, "my experience has been that almost any herb that is safe for an adult is safe for a child as long as the size and weight of the child are accounted for and the dosage is adjusted accordingly."[3]

There are a number of techniques for figuring out proper dosing:

Clark's Rule:

Take the weight of your child and divide it by 150. For example, if your child weighs 38 pounds you would divide 38 by 150 (38/150 = .253 or ¼) so your child would take ¼ of the adult dosage (White et al., 1998).[4]

Young's Rule:

Add 12 to your child's age and divide your child's age by this number. For example, for a 6 year old child: 6+12 = 18, then 6/18 = .3 from which you can calculate the fraction of the adult dosage to use. In this case, that would be 1/3 of the adult dosage.[5]

We have already done the math to come up with the following dosage recommendations and have based it on a 35-pound, medium-build child. You should adjust down or up depending on your child's weight and age. The exact dose for any given child should not be determined without the advice of your health care practitioner. Our suggestions here do not constitute medical advice or prescriptions and are purely educational in nature.

Aloe vera

- Topical: Use the gel from the inner side of the leaf. Slice a leaf in half and scoop out the soft gel for topical use. This can be done as often as desired.

- Important: The white, milky latex which is between the green part of the leaf and the clear gel, can be toxic-avoid using this.

Astragalus (*Astragalus membranaceus*)

- Root; immune supportive, antiviral, adaptogenic.

- Tea: 1 teaspoon dried root per 8–10 ounces of water. Place root in a cup, add boiling water and cover, allow to steep for fifteen minutes, strain before drinking. Optional: You can sweeten it with a little raw honey or add a squeeze of fresh lemon juice. This can be taken 3–5 times a day (4 ounces at a time for little ones).

- Glycerite: 10–30 drops in 2 ounces water up to three times a day.

- Astragalus and Elderberry is an excellent combination to have on hand and they mix well either as a tea or glycerite. For the glycerite, you can order an empty 4 ounces amber bottle and combine equal amounts of Astragalus and Elderberry glycerites and use together. Use 10–30 drops in 2 ounces water up to three times a day.

Barberry (*Berberis vulgaris*)

- Root; immune support, antiviral, antibacterial.

- Glycerite: 8–15 drops in 2 ounces water up to three times a day.

Burdock (*Arctium lappa*)

- Root; liver support, immune stimulating, anti-inflammatory.

- Tea: 1 teaspoon dried root per 8–10 ounces of water. Place root in a cup, add boiling water and cover, allow to steep for fifteen minutes, strain before drinking. Optional: You can sweeten it with a little raw honey or add a squeeze of fresh lemon juice. This can be taken 3–5 times a day (4 ounces at a time for little ones).

Coptis (*Coptis chinensis*)

- Root; antimicrobial, antiinflammatory, antioxidant.

- Glycerite: 8–15 drops in 2 ounces water up to three times a day.

Echinacea (*Echinacea angustifolia* and/or *Echinacea purpurea*)

- Whole plant; alterative (cleans the blood and restores normal function) antimicrobial, tonic.

- Tea: ¼–½ teaspoon dried plant. Place plant in a cup, add almost boiling water and cover, allow to steep for fifteen minutes, strain before drinking. Optional: You can sweeten it with a little raw honey or add a squeeze of fresh lemon juice. This can be taken 3–5 times a day (4 ounces at a time for little ones).

- Glycerite (1:2): 10 drops every 2–3 hours

- The secret to the effectiveness of echinacea is dosing frequently, every 2–3 hours.

Elderberry (*Sambucus nigra*)

- Berries; alterative, anti-histamine, reduces nerve pain, anti-oxidant, soothes GI tract, supports emunctories (channels of detoxification), reduces mucus, expectorant, immune supportive, antiviral.

- All parts of this plant may be used. However, for the purposes of this book, we are discussing the berries, which cannot be consumed when unripe. In addition, the use of the bark and root have to be supervised by a trained professional. That said, the dried berries are very safe and it is recommended that you purchase the dried berries to make tea and syrups.

- Tea: 1 teaspoon to 1 tablespoon dried berries. Place berries in a cup, add almost boiling water and cover, allow to steep for 15–20 minutes, strain before drinking. Optional: You can sweeten it with a little raw honey or add a squeeze of fresh lemon juice. This can be taken 3–5 times a day (4 ounces at a time for little ones).

- Glycerite: 10–30 drops in 2 ounces water up to four times a day.

- Elderberry and Astragalus is an excellent combination to have on hand and they mix well either as a tea or glycerite. For the glycerite, you can order an empty 4 ounces amber bottle and combine equal amounts of Astragalus and Elderberry glycerites and use together. Use 10–30 drops in 2 ounces water up to three times a day.

Elecampane (*Inula helenium*)

- Root; alterative (restores normal function), antiseptic, expectorant, relaxing, tonic.

- Tea: ¼–½ teaspoon root. Place root in a cup, add almost boiling water and cover, allow to steep overnight, warm and strain before drinking. Optional: You can sweeten it with a little raw honey or add a squeeze of fresh lemon juice. This can be taken 3–5 times a day (4 ounces at a time for little ones).

- Glycerite: 8–15 drops in 2 ounces water up to three times a day.

Garlic (*Allium sativum*)

- Bulb; reduces blood clotting, relieves GI upset, premier antimicrobial, reduces spasm, reduces external irritation, improves digestion, expectorant.

- Food: Best when it is eaten raw, but most little ones will not tolerate that well. Some ideas include: Add dried garlic to food, add freshly chopped garlic to teas and soups, in a garlic and onion syrup or garlic and ginger tea (see Recipes).

- Fluid extract: Kyolic Aged Garlic Extract, ⅛–¼ teaspoon in 2 ounces of water.

- Glycerite: 8–15 drops in 2 ounces water up to three times a day.

- As soon as fresh garlic is chopped and exposed to air, it begins to oxidize. The pre-chopped garlic in oil that you buy in the store does add flavor to food but has little to no medicinal value. The best way to utilize garlic medicinally is to buy it fresh, in bulb form, and only peel and chop right before you use it.

Ginger (*Zingiber officinale*)

- Root; pain reducer, antimicrobial, anti-inflammatory, anti-oxidant, reduces spasm, soothes GI tract, rubefacient (warms skin, reduces pain), very warming.

- Herbalists often caution the use of this herb with a high fever.

- Tea: ¼–½ teaspoon freshly grated root. Place grated root in a cup, add almost boiling water and cover, allow to steep for fifteen minutes, and strain before drinking.Optional: You can sweeten it with a little raw honey or add a squeeze of fresh lemon juice. This can be taken 3–5 times a day (4 ounces at a time for little ones). Tip: Store your ginger root in freezer because it grates more easily and preserves best in this way.

- Glycerite: 8–15 drops in 2 ounces water up to three times a day.

- As part of a garlic-ginger oxymel or garlic and ginger tea (see Recipes).

Goldenseal (*Hydrastis canadensis*)

- Root; immune support, antiviral, antibacterial.

- Glycerite: 8–15 drops in 2 ounces water up to three times a day.

Gotu kola/ Indian pennywort (*Centella asiatica*)

- Whole plant; adaptogen (restores normal function), fever reducer, reduces spasm, supports and heals nervous system, vulnerary (heals external tissue).

- Tea: ½–1 teaspoon dried plant per 8–10 ounces of water. Place plant in a cup, add almost boiling water and cover, allow to steep for 15 minutes, strain before drinking. Optional: You can sweeten it with a little raw honey or add a squeeze of fresh lemon juice. This can be taken 3–5 times a day (4 ounces at a time for little ones).

- Glycerite: 8–15 drops in 2 ounces water up to 3 times a day.

Hyssop (*Hyssopus officinalis*)

- Aerial parts; reduces spasm, antiviral, expectorant, relaxing, vulnerary (heals external tissue).

- Tea: ½–1 teaspoon dried plant per 8–10 ounces of water. Place plant in a cup, add almost boiling water and cover, allow to steep for 15 minutes and strain before drinking. Optional: You can sweeten it with a little raw honey or add a squeeze of fresh lemon juice. This can be taken 3–5 times a day (4 ounces at a time for little ones).

- Glycerite: 8–15 drops in 2 ounces water up to 3 times a day.

Lavender (*Lavandula angustifolia*)

- Flowers; antimicrobial, antifungal, pain reliever, reduces spasm.

- Tea: ½–1 teaspoon dried flowers per 8 to10 ounces of water. Place flowers in a cup, add almost boiling water and cover, allow to steep for fifteen minutes, strain before drinking.Optional: You can sweeten it with a little raw honey or add a squeeze of fresh lemon juice. This can be taken 3–5 times a day (4 ounces at a time for little ones).

- Glycerite: 8–15 drops in 2 ounces water up to three times a day.

- Topical in essential oil form mixed with a carrier oil such as coconut oil.

Lemon balm (*Melissa officinalis*)

- Aerial parts; pain reliever, reduces spasm, antiviral, reduces anxiety, soothes the GI tract, calms and heals nervous system, relaxing.

- Tea: ½–1 teaspoon dried plant per 8–10 ounces of water. Place plant in a cup, add almost boiling water and cover, allow to steep for 15 minutes, strain before drinking. Optional: You can sweeten it with a little raw honey or add a squeeze of fresh lemon juice. This can be taken 3–5 times a day (4 ounces at a time for little ones).

- Glycerite: 8–15 drops in 2 ounces water up to 3 times a day.

Licorice (*Glycyrrhiza glabra*)

- Root; adaptogen (restores normal function), anti-inflammatory, anti-oxidant, reduces spasm, expectorant, liver protective.

- Tea: ½–1 teaspoon dried root per 8–10 ounces of water. Place root in a cup, add almost boiling water and cover, allow to steep for fifteen minutes, strain before drinking. Optional: You can sweeten it with a little raw honey or add a squeeze of fresh lemon juice. This can be taken 3–5 times a day (4 ounces at a time for little ones).

- Glycerite: 8–15 drops in 2 ounces water up to three times a day.

Linden tree (*Tilia europa*)

- Flowers; reduces anxiety, reduces spasm, relaxing.

- Tea: ½–1 teaspoon dried flowers per 8–10 ounces of water. Place flowers in a cup, add almost boiling water and cover, allow to steep for fifteen minutes, strain before drinking. Optional: You can sweeten it with a little raw honey or add a squeeze of fresh lemon juice. This can be taken 3–5 times a day (4 ounces at a time for little ones).

- Glycerite: 8–15 drops in 2 ounces water up to three times a day.

Lomatium (*Lomatium dissectum*)

- Root; antibacterial, antifungal, antiseptic, antitussive, antiviral, expectorant, nutritive.

- Tea: ½–1 teaspoon dried root per 8–10 ounces of water. Place root in a cup, add almost boiling water and cover, allow to steep for fifteen minutes, strain before drinking. Optional: You can sweeten it with a little raw honey or add a squeeze of fresh lemon juice. This can be taken 3–5 times a day (4 ounces at a time for little ones).

- Glycerite: 8–15 drops in 2 ounces water up to three times a day.

Marshmallow root (*Althaea officinalis*)

- Root and Leaf; emollient (soothing to tissue), expectorant.

- Tea: ½–1 teaspoon dried leaves per 8–10 ounces of water. Place leaves in a cup, add almost boiling water and cover, allow to steep for fifteen minutes, strain before drinking. Optional: You can sweeten it with a little raw honey or add a squeeze of fresh lemon juice. This can be taken 3–5 times a day (4 ounces at a time for little ones).

- ◆ Glycerite: 8–15 drops in 2 ounces water up to three times a day.

Mullein (*Verbascum thapsus*)

- ◆ Foliage part; pain relieving, antimicrobial, reduces spasms, expectorant, relaxing and stimulating.

- ◆ Tea: ½–1 teaspoon dried foliage per 8–10 ounces of water. Place leaves in a cup, add almost boiling water and cover, allow to steep for fifteen minutes, strain before drinking. Optional: You can sweeten it with a little raw honey or add a squeeze of fresh lemon juice. This can be taken 3–5 times a day (4 ounces at a time for little ones).

- ◆ Glycerite: 8–15 drops in 2 ounces water up to three times a day.

- ◆ Poultice: see below.

Nettles (*Urtica dioica*)

- ◆ Leaf; anti-inflammatory, antihistamine.

- ◆ Tea: ½–1 teaspoon dried leaves per 8–10 ounces of water. Place leaves in a cup, add almost boiling water and cover, allow to steep for fifteen minutes, strain before drinking. Optional: You can sweeten it with a little raw honey or add a squeeze of fresh lemon juice. This can be taken 3–5 times a day (4 ounces at a time for little ones).

- ◆ Glycerite: 8–15 drops in 2 ounces water up to three times a day.

> **Caution: Sometimes people can have a mild reaction to nettles. It is wise to test it in small amounts befor using large amounts before using large amounts.**

Oats (*Avena sativa*)

- ◆ Aerial parts; nervous system restoration, highly nutritive.

- ◆ Glycerite of the milky oat seeds: 8–15 drops in 2 ounces water up to three times a day.

- Tea: 1 teaspoon oatstraw per 8–10 ounces of water. Place straw in a cup, add almost boiling water and cover, allow to steep for fifteen minutes, strain before drinking. Optional: You can sweeten it with a little raw honey or add a squeeze of fresh lemon juice. This can be taken 3–5 times a day (4 ounces at a time for little ones).

- Soaking baths: is a great herb to add to a soaking bath. See instructions for Soaking Baths in the Hydrotherapy section.

Oregon grape root (*Mahonia aquifolium*)

- Root; antimicrobial.

- Glycerite: 8–15 drops in 2 ounces water up to three times a day.

Osha (*Ligusticum porteri*)

- Root; antimicrobial antiseptic, reduce spasms.

- Glycerite: 8–15 drops in 2 ounces water up to three times a day.

Green tea (*Camelia sinensis*)

- Leaves; antimicrobial, antioxidant, immune stimulant, stimulant (use during the day).

- Tea: ½ teaspoon dried leaves per 8–10 ounces of water. Place leaves in a cup, add almost boiling water and cover, allow to steep for fifteen minutes, strain before drinking. Optional: You can sweeten it with a little raw honey or add a squeeze of fresh lemon juice. This can be taken 3–5 times a day (4 ounces at a time for little ones).

- Glycerite: 8–15 drops in 2 ounces water up to three times a day.

Pleurisy (*Asclepias tuberosa*)

- Root; relaxing expectorant.

- Tea: ½ teaspoon dried root per 8–10 ounces of water. Place root in a cup, add boiling water and cover, allow to steep for fifteen minutes, strain before drinking. Optional: You can sweeten it with a little raw honey or add a squeeze of fresh lemon juice. This can be taken 3–5 times a day (4 ounces at a time for little ones).

♦ Glycerite: 8–15 drops in 2 ounces water up to three times a day.

Sage (*Salvia officinalis*)

♦ Leaves; antimicrobial.

♦ Tea: ½ tablespoon fresh sage leaves or ½ teaspoon dried sage per 8–10 ounces of water. Place sage leaves in a cup, add boiling water and cover, allow to steep for fifteen minutes, strain before drinking. Optional: You can sweeten it with a little raw honey or add a squeeze of fresh lemon juice. This can be taken 3–5 times a day (4 ounces at a time for little ones).

♦ Glycerite: 8–15 drops in 2 ounces water up to three times a day.

Thyme (*Thymus vulgaris*)

♦ Leaves; antimicrobial.

♦ Tea: ½–1 teaspoon fresh or ¼–½ dried thyme leaves per 8–10 ounces of water. Place thyme leaves in a cup, add boiling water and cover, allow to steep for fifteen minutes, strain before drinking. Optional: You can sweeten it with a little raw honey. This can be taken 3–5 times a day (4 ounces at a time for little ones).

♦ Glycerite: 8–15 drops in 2 ounces water up to three times a day.

♦ Suggestion: Use in steam inhalations or vaginal steaming.

Supplements

In general, the vitalistic naturopathic approach supports obtaining nutrients through one's diet. The following information is not recommended for a daily nutrient intake, but rather is a guide to using supplements during an acute illness. We highly recommend working with a holistic nutritionist or a naturopathic doctor to identify and develop strategies to create and maintain a general state of health.

Active Hexose Correlated Compound (AHCC)

Best used as a powder mixed in with food. Buying AHCC powder is the most convenient way to purchase it. Simply mix with food when ready to administer.

- Infants less than one year old: 500 mg per day

- Children 1–4 years old: 500–1000 mg per day

- 4–8 years old: 1000–1500 mg per day

- 9–13 years old: 1500–2000 mg per day

- 14–18 years old: 2000–3000 mg per day[6]

Beta-carotene

Best taken in a capsule.

- The following dose is only recommended for HPV infection and for up to three months: 150,000 IU per day

Carnosine

Best used as a powder in apple or pear sauce.

- Infants less than one year and up to three years old: 400 mg per day

- Children three years and older 400 mg twice a day[7]

D-Ribose

Best used as a powder in apple or pear sauce.

- Infants less than one year old: 250 mg per day

- Children 1–4 years old: 250–500 mg per day

- 4–8 years old: 500–1500 mg per day

- 9–13 years old: 1500–3000 mg per day

- 14–18 years old: 5–10 g per day[8]

Essential Fatty Acids: Omega 3's: alpha linolenic acid (ALA), Eicosapentaenoic acid (EPA), Docosahexaenoic acid (DHA)

Best taken as a liquid with a fatty meal.

- Infants less than one year: 500 mg per day

- Children 1–3 years old: 700 mg per day

- 4–8 years old: 900 mg per day

- 9–13 years old: 1200 mg per day

- 14–18 years old: 1600 mg per day

Lecithin

See Phosphatidylcholine

Lysine (L-lysine)

Best taken as a powder mixed into apple or pear sauce.

- For children, 10 mg per pound of body weight is the place to start. Multiplying 10 mg by a child's weight in pounds will get the correct dose. For example, if a child weighs 35 pounds, multiply 10 x 35 = 350; 350 mg is the correct dose.

- If a child is thirteen years old and older, the recommended dose for adults (12 mg per kg body weight per day) is an appropriate dose. Always speak with your child's pediatrician about the appropriate use of lysine for your child.[9]

Magnesium glycinate

Best taken as a liquid.

- Infants six months and younger: 30 mg per day

- Infants 6 months-1 year: 50 mg per day

- Children 1–3 years old: 75 mg per day

- 4–8 years old: 150 mg per day

- 9–13 years old: 250 mg per day

- 14–18 years old: 300 mg per day

Mushrooms

Best taken as a liquid glycerite or powder in apple or pear sauce.

- Suggested formula should contain: chaga (*Inonotus obliquus*), cordyceps (*Ophiocordyceps sinensis*), reishi (*Ganoderma lucidum*) and shiitake (*Lentinula edodes*)

- Dose: 10–30 drops twice a day in 1–2 ounces of water.

N-acetyl cysteine (NAC)

Best taken as a powder mixed into apple or pear sauce. Buying NAC capsules is the most convenient way to purchase it. Simply open the capsule and mix it with food when ready to administer.

- Infants six months and younger: 250 mg per day

- Infants 6 months-1 year: 250 mg per day

- Children 1–3 years old: 300 mg per day

- 4–8 years old: 300–600 mg per day

- 9–13 years old: 600–1200 mg per day

- 14–18 years old: 600–1800 mg per day

Phosphatidylcholine

Best taken as a liquid.

- Infants six months and younger: 125 mg per day

- Infants 6 months-1 year: 15 0mg per day

- Children 1–3 years old: 200 mg per day

- 4–8 years old: 250 mg per day

- 9–13 years old: 375 mg per day

- 14–18 years old: 550 mg per day

Probiotics

Best taken as a powder in room-temperature milk or juice. Use a kids formula that has many different strains of lactobacillus and bifidus.

- Infants six months and younger (breastfeeding): cover nipple in probiotic powder twice a day before feedings

- Infants six months and younger (not-breastfeeding): ⅛ teaspoon in room temp milk twice a day

- Infants 6 months-1 year: ⅛ teaspoon twice per day

- Children 1–3 years old: ¼ teaspoon twice per day

- 4–8 years old: ½ teaspoon twice per day

- 9–13 years old: ¾ teaspoon twice per day

- 14–18 years old: 1 teaspoon 2–3 times per day (They can use a regular adult formula).

Vitamin A (retinol)

Mixed carotenoids is the best form to use.

- Vitamin A Flush: 5K units every three hours in coconut/almond/cashew milk for day 1, 10K every three hours day 2, 15K every three hours day 3, 18K every three hours day 4, then reverse days 5–8 until typical maintenance dose is achieved. Do not do this in the case of meningitis and/or if there is any encephalitis (brain swelling). In addition, it is best to work with a properly trained naturopathic doctor when using this therapy.

Vitamin B12 (Methylcobalamin)

The most absorbable form to use is methylcobalamin.

- B12 is best taken as a liquid or a sublingual tablet (this form is dependent on a child's ability to hold a tablet under the tongue).

- Infants less than 1 year old: 500 mcg per day

- Children 1–4 years old: 1000 mcg per day

- 4–8 years old: 1500 mcg per day

- 9–13 years old: 2000 mcg per day

- 14–18 years old: 2500 mcg per day

Vitamin C

- The best form to use is a whole food based vitamin C

supplement. It is best taken as a liquid, powder or chewable tablet (depending on child's ability to chew a tablet).

♦ 250–500 mg every two hours for two days. Lower doses with younger children. After two days, continue dose three times a day for three days. If child needs further support continue dose twice a day until child has recovered from illness.

♦ Do not use if diarrhea is present unless directed by your doctor.

Vitamin D3

Best taken as a liquid with a fatty meal. It is best used on a short term basis only during time of illness.

♦ Infants less than 1 year old: 400–500 IU per day

♦ Children 1–4 years old: 800–1000 IU per day

♦ 4–8 years old: 1200–1500 IU per day

♦ 9–13 years old: 1500–1600 IU per day

♦ 14–18 years old: 2000 IU per day

Zinc

Best taken as a chewable or a sublingual tablet (this form is dependent on a child's ability to hold a tablet under the tongue). These doses should only be taken for a short period of time since long term high dose intake of zinc can throw off the body's zinc-copper balance.

♦ Infants less than one year: 5 mg per day

♦ Children 1–3 years old: 5–10 mg per day

♦ 4–8 years old: 15 mg per day

♦ 9–13 years old: 15–25 mg per day

♦ 14–18 years old: 15–30 mg per day

Recipes

It is particularly important to use organic meats and whenever possible locally sourced organic produce in the following recipes. Additionally, we recommend you cook in cast iron, stainless steel, ceramic or glass pots and avoid aluminum based cookware. Try to avoid heating or cooking with a microwave.

Broths and Soups

Bieler's Broth

Simmer the following in a covered pot until very soft:

- 2 medium zucchini, chopped

- Handful of fresh green beans

- 2 stalks of celery, chopped

- 2 potatoes, unpeeled, chopped

- 1 cup chopped carrots

- 1 cup any other available dark green vegetable (collards, chard, kale, etc.)

- 1 cup tops (beets, turnips, radish, etc)

- 1 and ½ quarts of water

Add cayenne, basil, oregano, plus other desired seasonings (except salt). Cover and cook slowly for 1–2 hours. Cool for 30 minutes, strain and drink only the broth. Drink 2 cups a day.

Bone Broth

It is particularly important to use organic chicken for this recipe.

Yields: 3 quarts | Prep time: 20 minutes | Cook time: 14 hours 30 minutes

Ingredients

- 3 pounds bone-in chicken parts and gizzards

- 12 cups filtered water

- 1 tablespoon apple cider vinegar

- 1 yellow onion, peeled and quartered

- 3 large carrots, cut into large dice

- 4 cloves garlic, smashed

- 2 stalks celery with leaves

- 2 bay leaves

- 1 teaspoon sea salt

- 1/2 teaspoon cracked black pepper

- 1 bunch fresh parsley

Directions

Place the water and chicken parts in a slow cooker and cook on high for 2 hours. Skim off any foam from the surface and remove the chicken. Pull the meat off the bones, and set the meat aside. Return the bones to the pot.

Reduce slow cooker to low. Add all the remaining ingredients, except the parsley, to the pot and cook on low for 12 hours or on high for 6 hours. Turn off the pot, skim the fat off the top, stir in the parsley, and cover for 30 minutes.

Strain the broth through a fine-mesh sieve or cheesecloth. Store in the refrigerator or freezer for later use. Scoop off any solidified fat before using.[10]

Immune Soup

Ingredients

Note before beginning: You will need a "make it yourself" large tea bag or some cheesecloth to contain the Astragalus and reishi mushroom.

- 8 cups (1.9 liters) water

- 1 tablespoon (15 ml) sunflower oil

- 1 medium onion, diced

- 1 bulb garlic (at least 10 cloves), minced
- 1 and 1/2 inch (3 and 1/2 cm) piece of fresh ginger root, finely grated
- 2 stalks celery, chopped
- 5 pieces sliced dried Astragalus Root
- 1 large reishi mushroom
- 2 cups fresh, sliced shiitake mushrooms
- 1 large reishi mushroom
- 2 cups chopped kale
- 2 medium carrots, chopped
- ½ teaspoon Cayenne powder
- 1 teaspoon salt (to taste)
- 1 teaspoon black pepper
- ½ teaspoon Miso (optional)

Directions

Place astragalus and reishi mushroom in a cheesecloth, set aside. Bring water to boil in large pot. While water is coming to a boil, heat sunflower oil in a skillet. Sauté garlic, onions, celery and ginger until soft and aromatic. Add contents of skillet to pot of water. Add shiitake, astragalus and reishi, kale and carrots. Simmer covered for two hours. Remove from heat, allow to sit for two more hours. Remove Astragalus and reishi mushrooms. Reheat. Add salt, pepper and cayenne powder to taste. Add miso if desired.

Beverages

Electrolyte drinks

- Lemon water: ¼ cup fresh squeezed lemon juice to 8–10 ounces of warm or cold water.
- Homemade electrolyte drink: ½ teaspoon raw sugar and a pinch

of sea salt, Himalayan salt or mineral salt in 8 ounces of filtered water. Stir and drink 1 to 3 cups per day.

Everyday Herbal Tea

Ingredients:

- ¼ cup Rose hips

- 1 cup Lemon balm (*Melissa officinalis*) dried leaf

- ¼ cup Elderberry (*Sambucus nigra*) dried berries

- ½ cup Oatstraw (*Avena sativa*) dried herb

- 8 cups water

Directions:

Place all ingredients in a large pot and cover. Heat on low until mixture starts to simmer. Remove from heat, leave pot covered and allow to cool for at least 2 hours to extract medicinal ingredients. Strain into a container with a lid and store in the fridge for up to 5 days. This can be served cold or warm. To serve this tea warm, gently heat to desired temperature. You can sweeten with a little bit of raw honey or stevia if desired.

Garlic and Ginger Tea

Ingredients:

- ¼–½ teaspoon freshly grated ginger root

- 2–3 minced cloves garlic

- 1 ounce apple cider vinegar

- 1 teaspoon honey

- Fresh squeezed lemon juice to taste (optional)

- 16 ounces water

Directions:

Place grated ginger root and minced garlic in a container with lid. Add boiling water and cover. Allow to steep for 20 minutes. Cool and strain before drinking. Just before drinking, stir in apple cider vinegar and honey. Add a squeeze of fresh lemon juice, if desired.

Oxymel

Ingredients

- 1 bulb garlic, minced. *Do not use the pre-peeled and minced garlic sold in stores as this has already begun oxidizing.*

- 4 cups water

- ¼ cup raw honey

- ¼ cup apple cider vinegar

Directions

Peel and mince garlic cloves. Add to the water in a large pot with a cover, heat to boiling and boil until garlic is very soft, about 20 minutes. Remove from heat and allow to cool at least 1 hour. Add the honey and vinegar, mix well. Store in the refrigerator up to 5 days. Gently reheat on the stove before drinking. ½–1 cup per day.

Optional: can add 1 tablespoon finely minced fresh ginger root to make a Garlic and Ginger oxymel.

Caution: Do not use in respiratory illnesses where the temperature is greater than 103 degrees.

Turmeric Milk

Combine and heat up the following ingredients:

- 8 ounces coconut, cashew or almond milk

- ½ teaspoon turmeric

- dash of cinnamon

- dash of ginger

The longer it is heated the stronger the taste will be. Sweeten with raw honey if desired.

Syrups

Garlic and Onion Syrup

Ingredients:

- 1 small onion, sliced

- 1–2 bulbs fresh garlic, chopped

- 1 cup raw honey

Directions:

Layer onion and garlic in a glass jar. Completely cover onion and garlic with honey. Allow to sit for 2 days. Strain, bottle and store in a cool, dark place.

- Dose: adult 1–2 tablespoons 3x per day; child ½–1 teaspoon 3x per day

Herbal Syrup #1

Ingredients:

- 4–5 tablespoons Thyme

- 1 tablespoon Licorice

- 5 tablespoons Elecampane

- 1 cup Mullein

- ½ cup Coltsfoot

- 2–3 tablespoons Sundew (Drosera)

- Water

- Raw honey (for children over 1 year of age)

Directions:

Put herbs into pot and cover with 2 liters of water. Bring to a boil, then simmer until it is reduced to 1/3 its original volume. Strain out herbs and continue to simmer down to 1 liter liquid. Sweeten if desired. Give about 1 tablespoon per dose, 1 teaspoon for an infant. Can be frozen into ice cubes and sucked or crushed. Nursing mothers can take this as well and your child will get the benefit through breastmilk. This recipe can be doubled.[11]

Hydrotherapy

Constitutional Hydrotherapy

This treatment will typically be done at a naturopathic doctor's office, since it requires the use of a sine machine. However, this treatment can be done at home if parents are trained by their naturopathic doctor and they purchase a sine machine.

Supplies:

- 1 large bowl filled with cold water
- 1 large bowl filled with hot water
- 5 towels
- 1 wool blanket
- 2 sponge pads for sine wave
- 1 sine machine
- 1 massage table

Directions:

Lay wool blanket over massage table with more of the blanket on one side than the other. Have child lay face up on the blanket with arms at sides.

Fold blanket over legs up to waist.

Place sponge pads bilaterally between T5 and T6 alongside the spine.

Submerge two towels in hot water (alternately, can run towels under hot tap water), completely wring out excess water and place over chest and abdomen of child. Cover child with blanket and wait 5 minutes.

While the child is resting with the initial hot towels, prepare two additional towels, one hot and one cold towel. Submerge each in a tub of the corresponding temperature water and completely wring each one out before use.

After 5 minutes, uncover the child's chest and abdomen. Place the hot towel over the chest and abdomen for a moment then switch it for the cold towel. Immediately cover the child with the blanket. Turn on the sine machine to the lowest settings until the child feels gentle muscle contractions. The muscle contractions should not exceed the child's comfort level, i.e., this should not be painful. Leave the cold towel on for 10 minutes. You can add an additional blanket(s) to warm the child if they feel chilled.

After 10 minutes, turn off the sine machine, uncover the chest and abdominal area, and remove the wet towel.

Change the placement of the sponge pads with one pad around T12/ L1 area and the other over the solar plexus (mid-stomach area). Cover the child up with the blanket, turn up the sine machine to the child's comfort level and allow the child to lay for 10 minutes.

While the child is going through this next phase, prepare two hot towels.

After 10 minutes, uncover the child, remove the pads and towel.

Have the child turn over and place two hot towels over the child's back. Cover the child's back with the wool blanket and leave hot towels on for 5 minutes.

While the child is going through this phase, prepare one hot towel and one cold towel.

After 5 minutes, uncover the child's back and change out the towels for a fresh hot towel. Keep the hot towel on for a moment, then change it out for the cold towel. Cover child with wool blanket and leave hot towel on for 10 minutes. This is the final step.

An important point of this therapy is to make sure the child is warm at the end of the treatment. If the child feels cold or cool at the end of the treatment, you can simply remove the last towel, add another blanket and let the child sleep.

Systemic (Full body) hydrotherapy

This is a treatment that alternates hot and cold towels along with a full body blanket wrap. It is done by leaving the hot towel in place for 5 minutes and the cold towel for 2 minutes in three rounds (hot-cold, hot-cold, hot-cold).

Supplies:

- ◆ 1 large bowl filled with cold water

- ◆ 1 large bowl filled with hot water

- ◆ 2 towels

- ◆ 1 wool blanket

Directions:

Lay wool blanket over bed. Have child lay in the middle of the blanket and keep arms at sides.

Fold blanket over child's legs up to waist and cover head.

Submerge one towel in hot water (alternately, can run towel under hot tap water), completely wring out excess water and place over chest and abdomen of child. Make sure towel is not too hot for child's skin. Cover child with blanket and leave hot towel on body for 5 minutes.

While the hot towel is on child, prepare the cold towel by either submerging it in cold water or running under cold water tap.

After 5 minutes, uncover child's chest and abdomen- keeping legs and head covered- and change out the towel with the cold towel. Cover up child and allow cold towel to stay in place for 2 minutes.

While the cold towel is on the child, prepare the hot towel by either submerging it in hot water or running it under the hot water tap.

At the end of 2 minutes, switch out the towel with a new hot towel. Repeat this process (hot-cold) two more times. End the treatment with a cold towel.

One of the critical steps of this therapy is changing out the towels as fast as possible to keep the effects of the treatment going. It is also important to make sure the child is warm at the end of the treatment. If the child feels cold or cool at the end of the treatment, you can either do one or two more cycles of alternating hot and cold towels to help regulate their body temperature or you can simply remove the last cold towel, add another blanket and let the child sleep.

This treatment can be done on a child of any age, including infants.

For infants, washcloths may be big enough to cover their chest and abdomen. Making sure the chest and abdomen are covered is vital to the effectiveness of the treatment.

Magic Socks

Historically, this hydrotherapy was called "Wet Sock Therapy." At some point, a marketing-savvy naturopath explained to young patients that the overnight drying of the socks was a "healing magic trick" and the name quickly evolved into "Magic Socks." Kids love it and it actually does work like magic to arrest the onset of mild colds and flus. Here's how:

When covered with wool, damp socks draw congestion from the head and work overnight to stimulate systemic circulation. This treatment reflexively decreases congestion in the upper respiratory passages, head and throat.

The socks will dry overnight as the body brings warm, fresh blood to the feet. This, in turn, invigorates the immune system and helps fend off acute illness. Magic Socks can be used nightly when any concern exists about the onset of an acute infection or illness and with any ongoing insomnia.

For best results, repeat treatment for three nights in a row or as instructed by your doctor. If your child develops a loss of sensation in their feet while using Magic Socks, remove the socks and check in with your doctor. Do not use this therapy with any condition that has resulted in loss of sensation or circulation to the feet unless first consulting with your doctor.

Steam Inhalations (Infusion Steam Tent)

Ingredients

- 3 liters of water

- Large pot

- Chosen essential oils or herbs

- Large towel

Directions

Bring 3 liters of water to a boil in a large pot. Add a large handful of dried herb (preferably organic) or 2–3 drops of indicated essential oil. If you are using dried herbs, cover pot and allow to steep for 10 minutes. Then have your child sit with his or her face leaning over the pot, covering his or her head with a large bath towel.

Encourage your child to breathe in the steam for 10 minutes or longer. Duck your own head under the towel at first to ensure the steam is not too hot and won't burn the face or lungs. Use the steam tent a few times a day and at night before bed during acute periods of discomfort. This therapy is reported to bring great relief to the misery of whooping cough. Keep the eyes closed while inhaling the steam.[12]

For young children, create a blanket fort (e.g. a blanket draped between two chairs) and sit with them to make sure they are not burned by the hot water creating steam in the enclosed space. You also can place the steaming water in a small room, e.g. the bathroom, and have your child breathe in the steam. You can read a book or rock your child while he or she is breathing in the steam.[13]

Soaking Baths

- Herbal Baths: For most herbal baths, 1–2 cups of fresh or dried herb, is sufficient. The biggest challenge is keeping the tub from becoming a mess! One of the easiest things to do is use an extra large tea bag that you can fill with your own herbs. To make sure the oils of the plant are released, fill the tub with very hot water and allow to cool to a comfortable temperature. Soaking 15–20 minutes is a good rule of thumb to follow.

- Oat (*Avena sativa*) Bath: ½ cup finely ground oats, ¼ cup baking soda (pH balancer) and 2 tablespoons olive oil. Soak 15–20 minutes. The tub will be very slippery, so clean it thoroughly after bath.

- Epsom Salt Bath: Add 2 cups of Epsom Salt to warm water in a standard-sized bathtub. Double the Epsom Salt for an oversized garden tub. Soak 15–20 minutes.

  *Note:*The benefits of Epsom salt aren't just folklore. Numerous studies have demonstrated the profound and wide-ranging benefits of magnesium and sulfate, the two major components of Epsom Salt. Magnesium is the second-most abundant element in human cells and the fourth-most important positively charged ion in the body, so it's little wonder this low-profile mineral is so vital to good health and well being. Magnesium, also helps to regulate the activity of more than 325 enzymes and performs a vital role in orchestrating many bodily functions, from muscle control and electrical impulses to energy production and the elimination of harmful toxins.

Vaginal Steam

Boil water and pour over herbs in bowl (blend of oregano, thyme, basil and rose in equal parts). Place bowl underneath seat with hole in center (alternatively can place bowl on floor and squat over bowl but legs can tire out quickly this way). Wrap towel over lower back and drape over legs to capture steam in vaginal area. Make sure steam is not too hot. Sit over steam for 20–30 minutes. Can be done 2–3 times per week.

Physical Medicine

Chest Percussion

This is a massage technique where the sides of the hands quickly tap on your child's back to promote circulation in the lungs. Tap firmly and swiftly up and down your child's back for 5–7 minutes. Your child's skin may become slightly pink or red. This is a good sign letting you know blood is circulating. Most kids will enjoy this massage if it is not done too firmly and if they are not experiencing pain with coughing.

Craniosacral Therapy

The human body is naturally equipped with the ability to heal itself, and craniosacral therapy is one way of boosting your body's natural defenses. This therapy is a non-invasive, light touch method. The technique uses pressure (about the weight of a nickel) to remove restrictions within the craniosacral system. This system is closely connected to the central nervous system and is comprised of the membranes and fluid that surround the brain and spinal cord. Craniosacral therapy is a way to gently adjust the rhythm of the craniosacral fluid by eliminating barriers that can occur in the form of tightened body tissues, often caused by stress. Such barriers can cause tension and prevent optimal functioning of the nervous system. There are some excellent resources for learning how to do this and we have included them in the Resource section.

Dry Skin Brushing

Use a natural bristle brush (commonly available in most health food, drug and department stores for $5–$10). While not necessary, a long handle makes reaching all areas of the body easier. Brush before a shower or bath. Always brush towards the heart, using long, soft strokes, following the flow of the lymph and circulatory systems. Cover all areas of the skin. For areas such as the back, armpits, abdomen and both sides of the chest use a few clockwise strokes followed by a few counterclockwise strokes. Avoid any areas of the body where rash or broken skin is present.

Gargles

- Saltwater Gargle: For sore throat, make a warm salt water solution (12 ounces of warm water with 1 teaspoon of salt) and add 1–3 drops of essential oil (1 drop for children under 6 years of age). Gargle and spit the warm saline and tea tree mixture. Repeat every 2–3 hours.[14]

- Garlic Gargle: 4 cloves minced garlic in 2 ounces boiling water. Steep for 15 minutes, strain and gargle.

- Saltwater and Colloidal Silver Gargle: 8 ounces water + 1 teaspoon salt + 15 drops colloidal silver.

Massage

Massage includes many different types of hands-on techniques to promote circulation of blood and lymph through the tissues. In addition, massage is relaxing to children and human touch is healing. Children appreciate being touched by a loved one as it is time for bonding and feeling cared for.

When massaging a child, keep in mind that whereas someone with muscle tension may like and prefer deeper massage techniques, ill children are more likely to prefer light strokes over their back, on their arms and/or legs.

Using light pressure with your fingertips or thumbs, start with circular movements at your child's feet and work up the legs. Similarly, circular movements with light pressure can be used from the hands and worked up the arms. Moving towards the heart is helpful since it assists moving lymph in the direction of metabolic waste removal. Using a flat hand, across or up and down the back is soothing to a child.

Light pressure does not require using creams or lotions. If desired, using a food-based oil like olive, avocado or coconut oil are good options.

Children's skin is so thin that everything is easily absorbed.

Microcurrent Electrical Stimulation

Microcurrent electrical stimulation is the use of electrical stimulation to support enhanced cellular function. The treatment is based on the understanding that each body tissue has a specific frequency at which it normally exists. Electrodes are placed in appropriate areas where more electrical conduction is desired. Usually, water or a conducting gel is used to allow the signal to move through the body. Since the current is so small, people rarely feel any movement. Multiple treatments are usually necessary for the desired outcome.

Many companies have these machines available. Each of them have their own settings for treating conditions with inflammation, irregular cell growth cycles and pain. These machines are available to licensed practitioners. Treatments should be conducted by a practitioner trained in using this type of physiotherapy.

Poultices, Packs and Rubs

Burdock (*Arctium lappa*) Poultice

You can use fresh or dried Burdock root but it is easier to use dry. If you use fresh root, macerate (chop it up into a paste). If you use dry herb or powder, add just enough hot water to moisten and make a paste. Spread the paste evenly over the desired area. Wrap with gauze or muslin. Leave on for 10–15 minutes. Rinse well when finished.

Castor Oil Chest Rub

Pour about a nickle size castor oil over chest and rub it over your child's chest. You can also rub the oil over the abdomen if you have leftover oil. Castor oil can break up inflammation.

Castor Oil Pack

This treatment is designed to improve the functioning of your liver and to support this organ as it does one of its primary jobs: cleaning toxins from the body.

Materials Needed

- Plastic wrap

- Heating pad or hot water bottle

- Castor oil (cold pressed is preferred)

- Flannel cloth (cotton or wool)

- Baking soda (for cleaning up afterward)

- Bath towel (if using the non-heat method- see below)

- 2-3 safety pins (if using the non-heat method; see below)

Preparations

- Fold/cut flannel cloth into 3-4 layers thickness, about 6x6 inches in size

- Cut a piece of plastic wrap slightly larger than flannel

- Place plastic wrap on a hard surface and stack the 3-4 pieces of folded flannel on top

- Saturate flannel with castor oil (wet but not dripping)

- Place flannel on skin with plastic on top (plastic should cover flannel, flannel touching skin)

- Optional: An additional piece of plastic wrap can be used to wrap around the body thereby holding the entire dressing in place

Methods–Choose one of the following two methods:

With heat

- Place heating pad or water bottle on top of outermost layer of plastic wrap. If using heating pad turn to medium setting.

- Leave in place for 1-2 hours, but do not fall asleep with the pack in place.

- Heat promotes the absorption of castor oil and relaxes the internal organs. Heat should not be used if there is an internal abscess or if appendicitis is suspected. Check with your doctor if unsure.

Without heat

- ◆ Use a bath towel wrapped around body part and use pins to hold it in place. Overlapping the towel will ensure the castor oil does not get all over you and the surface you are laying on.

- ◆ Castor oil pack can be left on overnight.

Cleaning Up

- ◆ When castor oil pack is finished, clean area with a solution of 2 teaspoons of baking soda in 1 quart water.

- ◆ The pack can be stored in a plastic container and reused several times. Make sure it remains saturated with castor oil before each use.

Chest/Foot Rubs

Essential oil rubs: Add a total of 3–4 drops of essential oils to one tablespoon of pure, organic vegetable oil. Mix and rub into the feet and chest. You also can apply some just below the nose to provide support for nasal congestion. Rotate the combination of essential oils you are using every 2–3 days, to avoid the skin becoming sensitized to the essential oils. For children under six years old, add 3–4 drops to 2 tablespoons of pure, organic vegetable oil. Repeat application 3–4 times a day.[15]

Cleavers (*Galium aparine*) Poultice

You can use fresh or dried cleavers. If you use fresh leaves, chop them up into a paste, If you use dry herbs or powder, then add just enough hot water to moisten and make a paste. Spread the paste evenly over the desired area. Wrap with gauze or muslin. Leave on for 10–15 minutes. Rinse well when finished.

Garlic Socks

Smash 1 clove of garlic in garlic press. Divide and wrap up into two small bundles of cheesecloth. Rub olive oil on soles of child's feet. Place garlic cheesecloth bundle over soles of feet and put socks on over cheesecloth bundles. Children weighing over 50 lbs can use one clove of garlic per foot.

Iodine Rub/ Chest Rub

Use a carrier oil such as coconut, olive, sweet almond or sunflower oil. Add ¼–4 teaspoons of oil into a small glass container. The amount to use depends on how large an area to which you are applying the iodine rub.

Add iodine:

- ¼ teaspoon oil, add 5 drops iodine

- ½ teaspoon oil, add 10 drops iodine

- ¾ teaspoon oil, add 15 drops iodine

- 1 teaspoon oil, add 20 drops iodine

Mix well with a toothpick or small stirring item and apply liberally. Can be repeated every 2–3 hours.

Recommended product: Illumodine (see Resources section for purchasing information)

Lavender-infused Oil

Ingredients

- 2 ounces Lavender flowers, fresh or dried

- 8 ounces of almond, sunflower or olive oil

- 1 small glass jar

- 1 small pot

Directions

- Sun-infused (slower): To infuse an oil, loosely fill a small glass jar with fresh (or dried) herb and cover completely with oil. Place on a ledge in the sun for at least a week. The longer it sits, the more potent it becomes. Use as often as needed.

- Heat-infused (faster): Place fresh or dried herb and oil (almond, sunflower or olive) in a small pot and put in thermometer. Heat to approximately 120 degrees and "cook" at this temperature for 1 hour, stirring every 15 minutes. Strain oil.

Mullein (*Verbascum thapsus*) Poultice

- 1 tablespoon dried mullein

- 1 cup boiling water

- Steeping ball

Add 1 tablespoon of mullein leaf to the steeping ball. Pour this into a cup and add boiling water in it. Let it steep for 10 minutes so the mullein's properties are released. In the mullein tea, soak a clean cloth and put it over the area with the swelling symptom within a few minutes. Apply this method 5–7 times every day for a week.

Mustard Pack

Ingredients

- 4 tablespoons flour

- 1–2 tablespoons dry mustard

- Water (lukewarm)

Directions

Mix the dry ingredients together then add the water to make a paste. The paste should be smooth and easily spreadable but not too thin so that it runs or is watery.

Take a clean cotton flannel and spread the paste evenly across top half (one side only), fold up the bottom half of the towel and apply to chest area. Do not apply paste directly to skin or it may cause blistering.

Cover with a fresh towel. Leave plaster on for up to 20 minutes. Remove immediately if skin turns deep red and is in danger of blistering. Some reddening is normal as heat and circulation is being drawn to the surface.

Remove poultice, wash skin with a warm cloth to remove any traces that may have seeped through, and dry.

Can be reapplied every 6 hours as needed. Do not use if there are allergies to mustard or if there is a fever present.

Onion Poultice/ Chest Pack

Ingredients

- 2–3 onions

- Large bowl

- ½ cup flour

- 2 tablespoons apple cider vinegar

- Cotton flannel cloth

Directions

Finely chop onions and steam for 10 minutes. Place in a large bowl. Add flour and apple cider vinegar to bowl. Mix well. Place the entire mash in a cotton flannel cloth. Fold flannel so mash is in the middle and place over chest. Cover with a towel. Rest with the poultice on for at least 20 or 30 minutes.

Plantain (*Plantago major*) Poultice

You can use fresh or dried Plantain. If you use fresh leaves, chop them up into a paste. If you use dry herb or powder, add just enough hot water to moisten and make a paste. Spread the paste evenly over the desired area. Wrap with gauze or muslin. Leave on 10–15 minutes, rinse well.

Suppositories and Salves

Antioxidant Suppositories/Salve

Supplies

- ½ teaspoon calendula powder

- ⅛ teaspoon vitamin A

- ½ teaspoon marshmallow (Althea officinalis) powder

- Thuja essential oil

- ½ cup cocoa butter (or alternately can use coconut oil)

- 1 suppository mold (if making suppositories)

- 1 small glass jar

- 1 double boiler

Directions

In a double boiler, melt ½ cup cocoa butter (coconut oil). Remove from heat.

When the cocoa butter is slightly warm, and before it starts to solidify again, add 10 drops of thuja essential oil, calendula and marshmallow powder and vitamin A oil (vitamin A oil is not needed if using coconut oil). Stir and immediately remove from heat.

- For suppositories: Pour into suppository molds and allow to cool. Place in a storage container and store in a cool, dry, dark area. Insert a suppository nightly for 6 nights a week. Take one night off per week. Continue for 3 months.

- For salve: Pour into a sterile glass jar and allow to cool before capping. Store in a cool, dry, dark area. Insert ½ teaspoon of the salve vaginally with a clean or gloved finger before bed. Insert nightly for 6 nights a week. Take one night off per week. Continue for 3 months.

Treatment at night is recommended because the suppository or salve will quickly melt and run out of the vagina if you are standing. If you are lying down, the salve or suppository will stay in contact with the cervix longer. We advise you discontinue treatment during menstrual cycle.

Tea Tree Essential Oil Suppository or Salve

Supplies

- Tea tree essential oil

- ½ cup coconut oil

- 1 small glass jar

- 1 double boiler

- Suppository Mold (if making suppositories)

Directions

In a double boiler melt ½ cup coconut oil. Remove from the heat.

When the coconut oil is slightly warm, and before it starts to solidify again, add 48 drops of tea tree essential oil. Stir and immediately remove from heat.

- ◆ For suppositories: Pour into suppository molds and allow to cool. Place in a storage container and store in a cool, dry, dark area. Insert a suppository nightly for a week. Take a break for a week. Insert nightly for a week. Continue alternating one week on, one week off for at least 2 months.

- ◆ For salve: Pour into a sterile glass jar and allow to cool before capping. Store in a cool, dry, dark area. Insert ½ teaspoon of the salve vaginally with a clean or gloved finger at night, before bed. Alternate one week on, one week off, for at least 2 months.

Treatment at night is recommended because the suppository or salve will quickly melt and run out of the vagina if you are standing. If you are lying down, the salve or suppository will stay in contact with the cervix longer.

Vitamin E Suppository

Softgel vitamin E capsules can be inserted vaginally without any additional preparation. Mixed tocopherol or alpha tocopherol softgels work well.

Insert one gel daily for 6 days. Take one day off. Continue for 3 months. Discontinue during menstrual cycle.

1 Gladstar, R. (2001). *Rosemary Gladstar's Family Herbal.* North Adams, MA: Storey Books

2 Justis, Angela. "Choosing Safe Herbs For Your Kids." The Herbal Academy. https://theherbalacademy.com/choosing-safe-herbs-for-your-kids (accessed February 1, 2017

3 Ibid

4 AHCC Research Blog. "Taking AHCC: What to Know when Using this Nutritional Supplement." info.ahccresearch.com. http://info.ahccresearch.com/blog/taking-ahcc-what-to-know-when-using-this-nutritional-supplement (accessed June 1, 2017).

5 A Guide to Nurtitional Supplements. "L-Carnosine Benefits, Side Effects and Dosage." nutritional-supplements-health-guide.com. http://www.nutritional-supplements-health-guide.com/l-carnosine-benefits.html (accessed June 1, 2017).

6 AHCC Research Blog. "Taking AHCC: What to Know when Using this Nutritional Supplement." info.ahccresearch.com. http://info.ahccresearch.com/blog/taking-ahcc-what-to-know-when-using-this-nutritional-supplement (accessed July 10, 2017).

7 Danielle Walker Against All Grain. "Chicken Stock (Bone Broth)." againstallgrain.com. https://againstallgrain.com/2014/03/03/chicken-stock-bone-broth (accessed February 1, 2016).

8 Dr. Will Taylor

9 Adapted from Thyme Infusion Steam Tent From Dr. Will Taylor

10 Dr. Judith Boice ND, LAc, FABNO

11 Dr. Judith Boice ND, LAc, FABNO

12 Dr. Judith Boice ND, LAc, FABNO

PART VII:
Resources

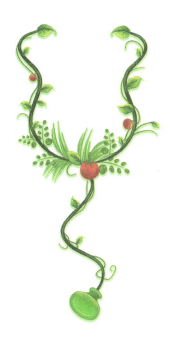

For Parents

Locating a Vitalistic Naturopathic Doctor

◆ Naturopathic Medicine Institute:
www.naturopathicmedicineinstitute.org

Physical Medicine

◆ Craniosacral at home training:
https://www.massagetherapyceu.com/course_details.php?cid=10

◆ Hydrotherapy at home

◆ http://www.care2.com/greenliving/thirteen-tips-for-using-hydrotherapy.html

◆ https://www.theguardian.com/lifeandstyle/2008/jul/06/healthandwellbeing.relaxation26

◆ Dr. Letitia Dick-Kronenberg:
https://www.youtube.com/watch?v=D4JecYJ53GY

◆ Lymphatic Massage:
http://www.massagetherapy.com/articles/index.php/article_id/1200/Lymph-Drainage-for-Detoxification-

◆ Massage:
http://www.liddlekidz.com/massage-your-child.html

Home Study Courses

◆ Complete Course Offerings at Vital Health:
https://www.vitalhealthpublishing.com/courses

◆ Green Medicine Chest Course with Dr. Boice:
http://www.drjudithboice.com/info/greenmedicinead4.html

◆ Homeopathic Home Practitioner Training with Eli Camp, ND, DHANP:
http://www.vitalhealthpublishing.com/courses

♦ Vaccination Series with Judith Thompson, ND:
http://www.vitalhealthpublishing.com/courses

Products

As parents look at different herbal formulas or supplements, it's important to remember that since herbs and natural supplements are new or unusual tastes for children, many companies add sugar, or sugar substitutes, to make their products taste good. Sugar has been shown to suppress normal immune function for up to five hours. Since many parents don't realize that 4 grams of sugar equals one teaspoon, they may inadvertently give their children a product with high amounts of sugar. The best way to avoid this is by reading labels before purchasing any products and paying attention to the amount of sugar. Also, contrary to what you may have heard, sugar substitutes aren't any better for health. We suggest avoiding those as well whenever possible.

If you currently work with a naturopathic doctor or other qualified holistic health professional, we recommend you discuss getting the recommended items below from them, as they may have their own favorite brands. If you would rather visit your local health food store or order online, we have provided our favorite non-practitioner level products.

Essential Oils

♦ Plant therapy:
http://amzn.to/2xksA7l

♦ Floracopeia:
http://amzn.to/2xkc1It

♦ Veriditas:
http://veriditasbotanicals.com/

♦ Neil's Yard Remedies:
http://amzn.to/2xjP6Nm

♦ Ameo:
http://amzn.to/2wuUsXe

♦ Imani:
http://www.imaninatural.com

- The Aromatherapist:
  https://www.thearomatherapist.com/

- Snow Lotus:
  http://amzn.to/2yopxJR

- Wellscent:
  https://well-scent.com/

- Essential Oil Wizardry:
  https://www.essentialoilwizardry.com/

- Nature's Symphony:
  http://nsaroma.com/

Herbs and Botanicals

- Avena Botanicals:
  https://www.avenabotanicals.com/

- Gaia Herbs:
  http://amzn.to/2ybQtLI

- Garden of Life: http://amzn.to/2fgJKfY

- Hawaii Pharm:
  https://www.hawaiipharm.com/?tracking=59bd7e52758dd

- Herb Pharm:
  http://amzn.to/2ynzpDk

- Host Defense:
  http://amzn.to/2xkti4v

- Mountain Rose Herbs:
  http://amzn.to/2xjG0jF

- Starwest Botanicals:
  http://amzn.to/2xPRQU8

Homeopathic remedies

- Bach Rescue Remedy:
  http://amzn.to/2jFlIfT

- Boiron:
  http://amzn.to/2fgfiSY

- Helios:
  http://amzn.to/2jHFkA7

- Hylands Homeopathics :
  ttp://amzn.to/2fhpMkY

- Washington Homeopathic:
  http://amzn.to/2fix3ky

Illumodine

- https://www.yogimedicine.com/product/illumodine-12-oz/

- https://www.drcousensglobal.com/illumodine-supplement-2-oz.html

Mushroom Formulas

There are many mushroom formulas available, these are the authors' favorites.

- Mycopotent by Biogenesis:
  http://amzn.to/2yontl5

- Myco Formula from Hawaii Pharm:
  https://www.hawaiipharm.com/tonic-of-emperor-alc-extract?tracking=59bd7e52758dd

- Host Defense MyCommunity Extract:
  http://amzn.to/2xkqjZT

- Host Defense Stamets 7:
  http://amzn.to/2xjBNMW

Supplements

- Biogenesis:
  http://amzn.to/2wug5qV

- Garden of Life:
  http://amzn.to/2xOWl1r

- Jarrow:
  http://amzn.to/2wETjYv

- Klaire Labs:
  http://amzn.to/2ybLOJD

- Nordic Naturals:
  http://amzn.to/2ynJ7Wg

- Priority One:
  http://amzn.to/2hgamue

- Pure Encapsulations:
  http://amzn.to/2ybH3Qo

- Standard Process:
  http://amzn.to/2yn7e7y

Teas and supplies

- Mountain Rose Herbs:
  http://amzn.to/2xjG0jF

Other Items

- Castor Oil:

    - Heritage Store Castor Oil:
      http://amzn.to/2xkkprk

    - Home Health Castor Oil:
      http://amzn.to/2xP6nQf

- Coconut Water:
  http://amzn.to/2xPmAox

- Colloidal Silver by Argentyn 23:
  http://amzn.to/2xuKNj4

- Dry Skin Brush:
  http://amzn.to/2fy99yh

- Home Health products:
  http://amzn.to/2wuOdmg

- Lozenges: Thayer's Lozenges:
  http://amzn.to/2xkrKY3 or
  Zand Organic Lozenges:
  http://amzn.to/2fhd711

- Thermometers (temple):
  http://amzn.to/2wueeSZ or http://amzn.to/2xkxaCn

Recommended Books, Articles and Websites

Books / Articles

- Aviva Romm, MD: Naturally Healthy Babies and Children: A
  Commonsense Guide to Herbal Remedies, Nutrition, and Health
  http://amzn.to/2wjZdCY

- Dana Ullman, CCH: Homeopathic Medicine for Children and Infants
  http://amzn.to/2wkBDGo

- James Green: The Herbal Medicine-Maker's Handbook: A Home
  Manual http://amzn.to/2wxIEP8

- Judith Boice, ND, LAc, FABNO: Green Medicine Chest http://amzn.
  to/2fbI0Va

- Juliette de Bairacli Levy: Nature's Children http://amzn.to/2x7lmSj

- Kate Birch, RSHom(NA), CCH, CMT: Vaccine Free: Prevention and
  Treatment of Infectious Contagious Disease with Homeopathy http://
  amzn.to/2yfmkMz

- Mary Bove, ND: An Encyclopedia of Natural Healing for Children
  and Infants http://amzn.to/2wjjicO

- Miranda Castro: Homeopathy for Pregnancy, Birth, and Your Baby's
  First Year http://amzn.to/2fcCuRU

- Rosemary Gladstar: Rosemary Gladstar's Family Herbal: A Guide
  to Living Life with Energy, Health, and Vitality: http://amzn.
  to/2xHgoyW

- Rosemary Gladstar: Rosemary Gladstar's Herbal Remedies for
  Children's Health http://amzn.to/2wjoA7T

◆ Thomas Kruzel, ND: The Homeopathic Emergency Guide: A Quick Reference Guide to Accurate Homeopathic Care http://amzn. to/2frMeVv

Websites

◆ Herbal use for children: https://theherbalacademy.com/choosing-safe-herbs-for-your-kids/

◆ Naturopathic Medicine Institute Public Facebook Group

For Practitioners

◆ Naturopathic Medicine Institute (NMI) http://www. NaturopathicMedicineInstitute.org. This may be one of the best resources for doctors treating unvaccinated children. The NMI exists to educate the public and medical practitioners about the principles and practice of naturopathic medicine. They strive to maximize the value of educational offerings by stressing practical knowledge for the healing arts primarily designed for naturopathic physicians and other allied professionals to facilitate their professional development.

◆ Homoeopathic leaders in pneumonia. Alfred Pulford. ISBN-13: 9788170212461 ISBN-10: 8170212464

◆ Quick Reference Rubrics on Warts by Dr. Nahida M. Mulla.

◆ NMI Book List: http://www.naturopathicmedicineinstitute.org/ bookstore/

◆ NMI Clinical Discussion Group, The Vital Conversation: The authors of this book are members of the NMI which is composed of many of the Elders of the Naturopathic Medical profession that were interviewed for this book. A discussion forum is available to naturopathic doctors who want to participate and who are NMI Associates.

References

Allen, H. C. 1978. *Keynotes and characteristics with comparisons of some of the leading remedies of the materia medica.* Wellingborough, Eng: Thorsons Publishers.

Allen, J. Henry, and Lutze, F. H. 1904. *The chronic miasms.* Chicago, Ill.

Allen, Timothy Field. 1880. *The encyclopedia of pure materia medica; Index.* New York, Philadelphia: Boericke & Tafel.

Birch, Kate. 2012. *Vaccine free prevention & treatment of infectious contagious disease with homeopathy: a manual for practitioners and consumers.* Kandern, Germany: Narayana Publishers.

Boice, Judith. 1996. *Pocket guide to Naturopathic medicine.* Freedom, Calif: Crossing Press.

Bove, Mary. 2001. *An encyclopedia of natural healing for children and infants.* Chicago: Keats Pub.

Boyle, Wade, and Andŕe Saine. 1993. *Lectures in naturopathic hydrotherapy.* East Palestine, Ohio: Buckeye Naturopathic Press.

"Colonic Enemas - A Naturopathic Treatment". 1998. *TOWNSEND LETTER FOR DOCTORS AND PATIENTS.* (180): 100.

Coulston, Ann M., Carol Boushey, and Mario G. Ferruzzi. 2013. *Nutrition in the prevention and treatment of disease.* Oxford: Elsevier/Academic.

Culpeper, Nicholas. 1867. *Culpeper's complete herbal: with nearly four hundred medicines, made from English herbs, physically applied to the cure of all disorders incident to man ; with rules for compounding them: also, directions for making syrups, ointments, &c., &c., &c.* London: Milner and Sowerby.

Dewey, Willis A. 1997. *Practical homeopathic therapeutics.* New Delhi: B. Jain.

Eizayaga, Francisco Xavier. 1991. *Treatise on homoeopathic medicine.* Buenos Aires: Ed. Marecel.

Gaby, Alan. 2011. *Nutritional medicine.*

Gaby, Alan. 2017. *Nutritional medicine.*

Genzlinger, Kelly, Kathy Erlich, and David Brownstein. 2012. *Super nutrition for babies: the right way to feed your baby for optimal health.* Beverly, MA: Fair Winds Press.

Green, James. 2000. *The herbal medicine-makers' handbook: a home manual.* Freedom, Calif: The Crossing Press.

Gupta, Ramji, O.P. Bhardwaj, and R.K. Manchanda. 1991. "Homœopathy in the treatment of warts". *British Homoeopathic Journal.* 80 (2): 108-111.

Hahnemann, Samuel. 1880. *Materia medica pura: in 2 vols.* London: Gould.

Hahnemann, Samuel, R. E. Dudgeon, and William Boericke. 2013. *Organon of medicine.* Kolkata: Modern Homœopathic Publication.

Hahnemann, Samuel, and Wenda Brewster O'Reilly. 1996. *Organon of the medical art.* Redmond, Wash: Birdcage Books.

Hering, Constantine, and C. G. Raue. 1879. *The guiding symptoms of our materia medica.* Philadelphia: American Homeopathic Publishing Society.

Hoffman, David. 1996. *Holistic herbal: a safe and practical guide to making and using herbal remedies.* Shaftesbury: Element Books.

Hudson, Allan. 2001. *Lymphatic drainage: therapy I.* Castlecrag, N.S.W.: Triam Press.

Karren, Keith J. 2010. *Mind/body health: the effects of attitudes, emotions and relationships.* San Francisco: Benjamin Cummings.

King, John, and Robert Stafford Newton. 1859. *The American Dispensary. By J.K. ... Fifth edition, revised and enlarged from "the American Eclectic Dispensary" [originally compiled by J.K. and R.S. Newton].*

Kruzel, Thomas. 1992. *The homeopathic emergency guide: a quick reference handbook to effective homeopathic care.* Berkeley, Calif: North Atlantic Books.

Lindlahr, Henry, and Jocelyn C. P. Proby. 1975. *Philosophy of natural therapeutics.* Saffron Walden: C.W. Daniel Co.

Lindlahr, Henry, and Victor Hugo Lindlahr. 1931. *The practice of nature cure.* New York city: The Nature cure library, Inc.

Lippincott, Rebecca Conrow, Howard A. Lippincott, and William G. Sutherland. 1943. *A manual of cranial technique.* Detroit: Academy of Applied Osteopathy.

Marohn, Stephanie. 2002. *The natural medicine guide to autism.* Charlottesville, VA: Hampton Roads Pub.

Marz, Russell B. 1999. *Medical nutrition from Marz: (a textbook in clinical nutrition).* Portland, Or: Omni-Press.

Mills, Simon, and Kerry Bone. 2000. *Principles and practice of phytotherapy: modern herbal medicine.* Edinburgh: Churchill Livingstone.

Murray, Michael T., Joseph E. Pizzorno, and Lara Pizzorno. 2005. *The encyclopedia of healing foods.* New York: Atria Books.

Neustaedter, Randall. 2002. *The vaccine guide: risks and benefits for children and adults.* Berkeley, Calif: North Atlantic Books.

Ody, Penelope. 1993. *The complete medicinal herbal.* New York, N.Y.: DK Publishing.

Parham, Peter. 2000. *The immune system.* New York: Garland Publishing.

Pitchford, Paul. 1996. *Healing with whole foods: oriental traditions and modern nutrition.* Berkeley, Calif: North Atlantic Books.

Pizzorno, Joseph E., and Michael T. Murray. 2013. *Textbook of natural medicine.* St. Louis, Mo: Elsevier/Churchill Livingstone.

Pizzorno, Joseph E., and Michael T. Murray. 1999. *Textbook of natural medicine.* Edinburgh: Churchill Livingstone.

Pulford, Alfred. 1985. *Homoeopathic leaders in pneumonia.* New Delhi: B. Jain Publishers.

Schroyens, Frederik. 2007. *The essential synthesis.* London: Homeopathic Book Publishers.

Sears, Robert. 2011. *The vaccine book: making the right decision for your child.* New York: Little, Brown.

Sensations As If A Repertory of Subjective Symptoms. 2002. Sydney, N.S.W.: B Jain Pub Pvt Ltd.

Sicile-Kira, Chantal. 2004. *Autism spectrum disorders: the complete guide to understanding autism, Asperger's syndrome, pervasive developmental disorder, and other ASDs.* New York: Berkeley Pub. Group.

Singh, Sapuran. 1987. *Hering's model cures.* New Delhi: Jain Publ.

Skowron, Jared M. 2009. *Fundamentals of naturopathic pediatrics.* Toronto: CCNM Press.

Spitler, Harry Riley. 1948. *Basic naturopathy; a textbook.* [Place of publication not identified]: American Naturopathic Assn.

Suen, R. M., and S. Gordon. 2003. "A Critical Review of IgG Immunoglobulins and Food Allergy - Implications in Systemic Health". *TOWNSEND LETTER FOR DOCTORS AND PATIENTS.* (241/242): 134-139.

*The New England Journal of Homeopathy*1992. Amherst, MA: New England School of Homeopathy Press.

Van Wyk, Ben-Erik, and Michael Wink. 2004. *Medicinal plants of the world: an illustrated scientific guide to important medicinal plants and their uses.* Portland: Timber Press.

Vasey, Christopher. 2009. *The naturopathic way: how to detox, find quality nutrition, and restore your acid-alkaline balance.* Rochester, Vt: Healing Arts Press.

Vermeulen, Frans. 1994. *Concordant materia medica.* Haarlem: Merlijn.

Vithoulkas, George. 1990. *Essence of materia medica.* New Delhi: B. Jain.

Webb, Geoffrey P. 2006. *Dietary supplements and functional foods.* Oxford: Blackwell Pub.

Wendel, Paul. 1951. *Standardized naturopathy.* Brooklyn, N.Y.: Wendel.

World Health Organization. 1999. *WHO monographs on selected medicinal plants.* Geneva: World Health Organization.

1957: A severe poliomyelitis epidemic occurred in Buenos Aires. The majority of homoeopathic doctors prescribed Lathyrus sativus as a preventative, and drug stores distributed thousands of doses to the public. None of those who used the prophylactic registered a case of contagion.

1975: During another poliomyelitis epidemic in Buenos Aires, 40,000 were given the homeopathic prophylactic Lathyrus sativus. None developed poliomyelitis.

About the Authors

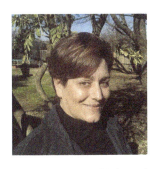

Eli Camp, ND, DHANP trained in naturopathic medicine at the Southwest College of Naturopathic Medicine in Tempe, AZ. She lectures across the country at numerous health conferences, public school districts and to the community in general regarding the topics of health and the practice of homeopathy. She serves as a preceptor for students from various fields of healthcare and as a mentor, consultant and coach to other Naturopathic Doctors to help them establish and become successful in private practice. Her memberships include the New Hampshire Association of Naturopathic Doctors (NHAND), the Oklahoma Association of Naturopathic Physicians (OKANP). the Homeopathic Academy of Naturopathic Physicians (HANP) and the Naturopathic Medicine Institute (NMI). In addition to membership, Dr. Camp served as Vice-President and President of NHAND, Treasurer of the FNPA and currently serves on the Board of the HANP and the NMI. She resides in Oklahoma with her 2 grandchildren, husband and 4-legged friend, Asia.

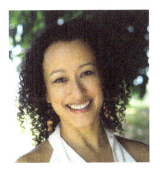

Judith Thompson, ND, trained in nutrition, herbal medicine, homeopathy, pharmacology and bio-energetics at the National University of Natural Medicine in Portland, Oregon. Her work combines naturopathic philosophy with modern science. Her years of delivering babies and caring for children nurtured her passion to see children grow up vitally strong. She has published articles nationally and internationally for medical journals and nutraceutical companies. She is the Vice President of the Florida Naturopathic Physicians Association and is a member of the Naturopathic Medicine Institute and the American Association of Naturopathic Physicians. She is a faculty member of Everglades University. She lives in Miami, FL, practices yoga and enjoys spending time in nature with her family, friends and dog.